Autonomic Nervous System in Old Age

....

Interdisciplinary Topics in Gerontology

Vol. 33

KARGER

Autonomic Nervous System in Old Age

Volume Editors   *George A. Kuchel, Farmington, Conn.*
Patrick R. Hof, New York, N.Y.

11 figures and 9 tables, 2004

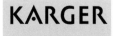

Basel · Freiburg · Paris · London · New York ·
Bangalore · Bangkok · Singapore · Tokyo · Sydney

··················
George A. Kuchel, MD FRCP
UConn Center on Aging
University of Connecticut Health Center
Farmington, Conn., USA

Patrick R. Hof, MD
Associate Professor, Kastor Neurobiology of Aging Laboratories
Dr. Arthur Fishberg Research Centre for Neurobiology
Mount Sinai School of Medicine
New York, N.Y., USA

Library of Congress Cataloging-in-Publication Data

Autonomic nervous system in old age / volume editors, George A. Kuchel, Patrick R. Hof.
    p. ; cm. – (Interdisciplinary topics in gerontology, ISSN 0074–1132 ; v. 33)
    Includes bibliographical references and index.
    ISBN 3–8055–7685–4 (hard cover : alk. paper)
    1. Autonomic nervous system–Pathophysiology–Age factors.   2. Autonomic nervous
system–Aging.   I. Kuchel, George A.   II. Hof, Patrick R.   III. Series.
    [DNLM: 1. Autonomic Nervous System–physiology–Aged.   2. Aging–physiology. WL
600 A939545 2004]
    HQ1060.I53 vol. 33
    [RC347]
    362.6 s–dc22
    [612.8'9]
                                                                          2003064038

    Bibliographic Indices. This publication is listed in bibliographic services, including Current Contents® and
Index Medicus.

    © Copyright 2004 by S. Karger AG, P.O. Box, CH–4009 Basel (Switzerland)
www.karger.com
    Printed in Switzerland on acid-free paper by Reinhardt Druck, Basel
    ISSN 0074–1132
    ISBN 3–8055–7685–4

Contents

Preface

In recent years, all western industrialized countries, and to a growing extent even many developed and developing Asian nations, have witnessed a remarkable growth in numbers of older people [1]. Future projections anticipate continued increases, particularly in numbers of individuals who are 85 years and older [1]. Although US statistics have indicated recent declines in disability trends [2], overall numbers of older individuals living with disability and functional dependence are likely to increase given projected increases in life expectancy [3]. For example, average life expectancy for women born today in the United States is nearly 80; for men, it is nearly 75 [1]. With these considerations in mind, many investigators have begun to pay increasing attention to identifying factors which may predict the transition from health and independence to disability and dependence in older individuals, eventually providing useful targets for interventions [3, 4].

Neurodegenerative disorders such as Alzheimer's and Parkinson's diseases are both common and important causes of cognitive and motor deficits in later life. Moreover, the presence of cognitive and motor deficits resulting from these disorders represents a major risk for the development of disability, dependence and need for institutionalization among older individuals [1]. Thus, it is not at all surprising that the central nervous system has received far more research attention than has the peripheral nervous system. Nevertheless, age-related changes and diseases involving the peripheral nervous system, particularly its autonomic elements, do frequently play determining roles in late life health and functional independence.

Homeostasis, the need for the body to maintain a constant internal milieu, was first defined by Claude Bernard in the mid 19th century [5]. In a 1932 book,

Walter B. Cannon clearly recognized that as the body ages its ability to maintain normal homeostasis in response to common challenges is altered [6]. In fact, many of the physiologic parameters discussed by Cannon – temperature, blood sugar and blood pressure – are all closely regulated by autonomic function and are discussed in some detail in this book. However, our understanding of autonomic system aging and its role in human health and disability has increased a great deal since the time of Bernard and Cannon.

Above all, modern clinical investigators typically study autonomic aging in healthy older individuals and are thus able to dissect the contribution being made by aging from that caused by disease. Such studies clearly indicate that while basal sympathetic activity increases with normative aging, there is evidence of considerable dysregulation in terms of the ability of the aging sympathetic nervous system to respond to a variety of challenges. Moreover, markers of elevated sympathetic activity appear to predict increased mortality among ill [7, 8], as well as community dwelling independent older individuals [9, 10].

Although many questions remain unanswered, recent conceptual and technological advances have provided both the clinician and investigator with much new information drawn from clinical, as well as basic research. In the following pages, investigators from several different disciplines discuss aging of the autonomic nervous system from a variety of perspectives. Given the fact that aging of the parasympathetic elements of the autonomic nervous system is not nearly as well understood as that of its sympathetic portions, greater emphasis has been placed on the latter. Some authors are basic scientists, while others are clinical investigators, yet efforts have been made by all to begin bridging the barriers between the two perspectives in a fashion that is meaningful to both.

In the first chapter, Dr. Schmidt discusses the major neuropathological and cellular changes that have been described during autonomic aging in both animal and human studies. Dr. Ford addresses the impact of physiologic changes involving the autonomic nervous system, but does so from the point of view of a clinical pharmacologist and clinician in describing the impact of age-related changes in autonomic function on responses to common medications. In Chapter 3, Drs. Attavar and Silverman discuss the impact of autonomic aging on cardiac performance and the management of common cardiac conditions. Drs. Bourke and Sowers focus their discussion on autonomic mechanisms involved in the regulation of blood pressure and the impact of age-related changes on the management of both hypertension and hypotension in older individuals. Aging is associated with specific deficits in the body's capacity to handle glucose and the role of autonomic aging in these changes is addressed by Drs. Madden and Meneilly. Many aspects of gastrointestinal function, particularly motility, are closely influenced by autonomic function. Drs. Pilotto, Franceschi, Orsitto and Cascavilla discuss the role of autonomic changes on gastrointestinal performance in late life. Urinary incontinence is a major cause of morbidity and disability in older individuals. Drs. Tannenbaum, Zhu, Ritchie and Kuchel provide an overview of age-related changes in the autonomic elements that closely regulate bladder performance and discuss their potential roles in maintaining continence in older women and men. As discussed by Drs. Beshay, Rehman and Carrier, both reproductive function and sexual performance decline in advanced age, with autonomic changes providing a contribution to both. The management of pain is a crucial element in improving the quality of life older patients and, as discussed by Drs. Lussier and Cruciani, autonomic changes are among the many important considerations needed to be brought into the assessment of an older individual in pain. Finally, the inability of many older individuals to appropriately regulate their body temperatures in response to both high and low extremes of environmental temperature is a major risk factor for death. Drs. McDonald, Gabaldón and Horwitz provide an excellent overview addressing a number of clinically important questions by highlighting key clinical and basic research studies.

Clearly, the years since Claude Bernard's first presentation of the concept of homeostasis and Cannon's comments regarding the influence of aging on these mechanisms have witnessed a tremendous growth in our knowledge. At the same time, the coming decade should lead to an even better understanding of this area. This will take place as more ambitious and well-defined clinical studies are undertaken and as the power of basic research is harnessed, particularly in terms of using genetically modified animals, with real efforts made to move or translate knowledge between the two fields.

George A. Kuchel, Farmington, Conn.
Patrick R. Hof, New York, N.Y

References

1   Guralnik JM, Ferrucci L: Demography and epidemiology; in Hazzard WR, Blass JP, Halter JB, Ouslander JG, Tinetti ME (eds): Principles of Geriatric Medicine and Gerontology. New York, McGraw-Hill, 2003, pp 53–76.
2   Fries JF: Measuring and monitoring success in compressing morbidity. Ann Intern Med 2003;139: 455–459.
3   Guralnik JM, Fried LP, Salive ME: Disability as a public health outcome in the aging population. Annu Rev Public Health 1996;17:25–46.
4   Fried LP, Tangen CM, Walston J, Newman AB, Hirsch C, Gottdiener J, et al: Frailty in older adults: Evidence for a phenotype. J Gerontol A Biol Sci Med Sci 2001;56:M146–M156.
5   Grande F, Visscher MB: Claude Bernard and Experimental Medicine. Cambridge, Mass., Schenkman, 1967.
6   Cannon WB: The aging of homeostatic mechanisms; in Cannon WB (ed): The Wisdom of the Body. New York, Norton, 1932, pp 202–215.

7   Semeraro C, Marchini F, Ferlenga P, Masotto C, Morazzoni G, Pradella L, et al: The role of dopaminergic agonists in congestive heart failure. Clin Exp Hypertens 1997;19:201–215.
8   Goldstein DS: Plasma catecholamines in clinical studies of cardiovascular diseases. Acta Physiol Scand Suppl 1984;527:39–41.
9   Seeman TE, McEwen BS, Singer BH, Albert MS, Rowe JW: Increase in urinary cortisol excretion and memory declines: MacArthur Studies of Successful Aging. J Clin Endocrinol Metab 1997;82: 2458–2465.
10 Reuben DB, Talvi SL, Rowe JW, Seeman TE: High urinary catecholamine excretion predicts mortality and functional decline in high-functioning, community-dwelling older persons: MacArthur Studies of Successful Aging. J Gerontol A Biol Sci Med Sci 2000;55:M618–M624.

Kuchel GA, Hof PR (eds): Autonomic Nervous System in Old Age.
Interdiscipl Top Gerontol. Basel, Karger, 2004, vol 33, pp 1–23

....

Age-Related Sympathetic Autonomic Neuropathology

Human Studies and Experimental Animal Models

Robert E. Schmidt

Division of Neuropathology, Department of Pathology and Immunology,
Washington University School of Medicine, Saint Louis, Mo., USA

Autonomic dysfunction is an increasingly recognized complication of human aging and, as a result of the rising mean age of the human population, has widespread ramifications for health care. Age-related autonomic neuropathy may produce clinical symptoms directly or result in subclinical disease, complicate therapeutic intervention in a variety of diseases (e.g., sympatholytic drugs in hypertension, aggressive insulin therapy in diabetes) or decrease the safety margin upon which superimposition of additional insults (e.g., diabetes) produce symptomatic disease. Early studies of the function and neuropathology of the autonomic nervous system in aged human subjects were largely anecdotal and often contradictory. However, recent systematic studies by a number of investigators have contributed substantively to the understanding of age-related autonomic dysfunction and its neuropathologic substrate. The development and use of animal models of human aging have begun to address pathogenetic mechanisms and intervention strategies in age-related autonomic dysfunction.

The Aging Human Autonomic Nervous System

Clinical Studies
Clinical studies [reviewed in ref. 1–5] support a role for age-related autonomic dysfunction in: (1) temperature regulation and sudomotor responses [6] which may lead to life threatening hypo- or hyperthermia; (2) bowel motility [7, 8], presenting as 'major gastrointestinal dysfunction' in 27% of one series of

hospitalized elderly [8, 9]; (3) visual abnormalities [10, 11]; (4) bladder function; (5) fat metabolism; (6) water and electrolyte regulation; (7) maintenance of blood pressure [12], and (8) cardiovascular reflexes [4, 10]. Cardiovascular dysfunction in aging is particularly complex and multifactorial, involving sympathetic [13] and parasympathetic [14] components as well as super-imposed endorgan impairment [15–19]. Exposure of the aged sympathetic nervous system to a variety of controlled experimental stresses may result in diminished [20] or unchanged [21] responses, or, surprisingly, produce an abnormally exaggerated [22, 23] (hyperadrenergic) response, observations hard to reconcile with the simple loss of sympathetic or parasympathetic ganglionic neurons. Alternatively, age-related autonomic dysfunction may involve inter-ference with the complex integration of autonomic functions within autonomic reflex pathways, which may take place in peripheral sympathetic ganglia [24] or at a number of other sites in the autonomic nervous system.

Neuropathology

The neuronal populations of aged human paravertebral superior cervical ganglion (SCG, fig. 1) and the prevertebral celiac (CG) and superior mesenteric (SMG) ganglia, are well preserved in aged human subjects, a result supported by a large autopsy series [25–27] and previous reports [28–30], although most human studies to date have not used unbiased stereologic counting techniques. Neuronal alterations described in aged human ganglia include decreased catecholamine fluorescence, accumulation of lipopigment and, in some studies [31], neurofibrillary tangles. The demonstration of perivascular and parenchy-mal lymphocytic infiltrates in postmortem sympathetic ganglia, widely inter-preted as evidence of an autoimmune process (e.g., diabetic autonomic neuropathy, idiopathic orthostatic hypotension), failed to correlate statistically with age, sex, diabetes or any other disease parameter and may largely reflect normal lymphocyte trafficking or a common aspect of the perimortem course [27].

In contrast to the apparent preservation of sympathetic ganglionic neurons, structural alterations in dendrites, axons and synapses have been consistently identified in aged human sympathetic ganglia [25–27, 32–36]. The hallmark pathologic alteration in aged sympathetic ganglia is neuroaxonal dystrophy (NAD), a distinctive axonopathy characterized by dramatic 5–30 μm axonal swellings (fig. 2). Dystrophic axons arise from delicate preterminal axons as a distal axonopathy or 'synaptic dysplasia' and displace the perikarya of principal sympathetic neurons or their primary dendrites [25]. Two types of dystrophic axons have been identified in aged human SMG [37]: most commonly, dys-trophic axons contain neurofilamentous aggregates with a specific immuno-phenotype; and, less frequently, tubulovesicular elements. Quantitative studies

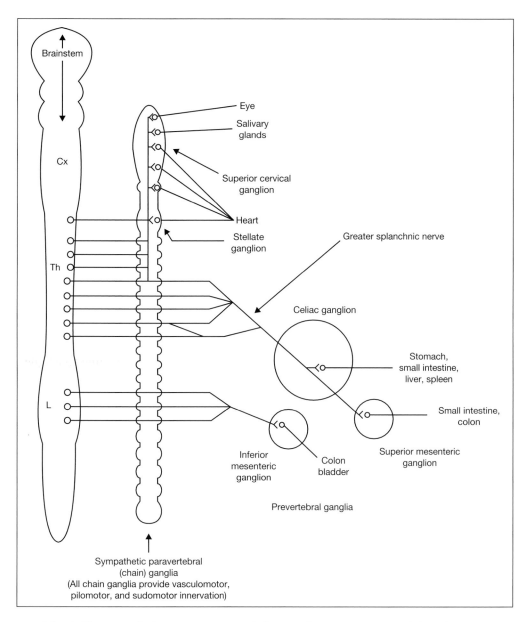

Fig. 1. The sympathetic nervous system. Only one of two paravertebral chains of ganglia are depicted. Figure modified from M.B. Carpenter: *Human Neuroanatomy*, ed 7, Baltimore, Williams & Wilkins, 1976, p 192.

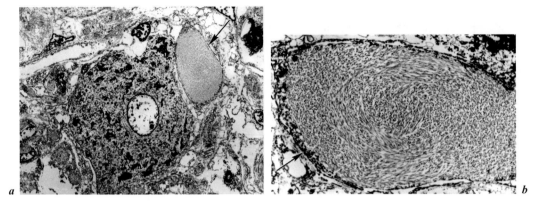

Fig. 2. Neuroaxonal dystrophy in aged human SMG. A markedly swollen dystrophic axon (*a*, arrow) is intimately applied to the perikaryon of a principal sympathetic neuron. Higher magnification demonstrates skeins of misoriented neurofilaments and a peripheral rim of dense core granules (*b*, arrow). *a* 2,740×; *b* 8,300×.

[27] have demonstrated a progressive increase in the frequency of NAD as a function of age (increasing particularly after the age of 60), gender (males had 3-fold more dystrophic axons than females) and diabetes (suggesting a shared pathogenetic mechanism between diabetes and aging).

Nerve terminals in the prevertebral ganglia represent the contribution of neurons originating in the spinal cord, dorsal root ganglia, parasympathetic nervous system, other sympathetic ganglia or as intraganglionic sprouts, and from retrogradely projecting intramural alimentary tract myenteric neurons, many of which have a distinctive neurotransmitter or neuropeptide signature. Dystrophic axons in aged human SMG are immunoreactive for tyrosine hydroxylase (TH), dopamine-β-hydroxylase (DβH) and neuropeptide Y (NPY) as well as trkA and p75[NTR] (high-affinity NGF and low-affinity neurotrophin receptors, respectively) but not substance P, GRP/bombesin, CGRP or enkephalins [25, 26, 38, 39]. This immunophenotype is most compatible with an origin of dystrophic axons from sympathetic neurons, intrinsic or extrinsic to the SMG. The total number of NPY-containing delicate nondystrophic axons and nerve terminals and perisomal DBH-containing processes of all sizes actually increased in the aged SMG, a result which may reflect intraganglionic collateral axonal sprouting as well as axonal regeneration. NPY released by sympathetic nerve terminals has been shown to inhibit presynaptic release of acetylcholine from intracardiac parasympathetic nerve terminals [40], a process which, if operative in sympathetic ganglia, could interfere with integration of nerve impulses derived from a variety of sources. Age-related loss of preganglionic neurons in the intermediolateral nucleus [41] may also contribute to the loss of subpopulations of axon terminals surrounding principal sympathetic neurons [29].

The neurofilaments (NF) which accumulate in dystrophic sympathetic nerve terminals of aged human SMG consist almost exclusively of extensively phosphorylated 200-kD NF-H epitopes [42]. Antisera directed against NF-L, NF-M and nonphosphorylated epitopes of 200-kD NF-H preferentially label sympathetic neuronal perikarya and principal dendrites and do not label dystrophic axons, evidence against the origin of NAD from principal dendrites or proximal perisomal portions of axons. Simultaneous immunolabeling of phosphorylated NF-H proteins (dystrophic axons) and MAP-2 protein (a marker for dendrites and cell bodies) also failed to demonstrate colocalization. Peripherin, a 58-kD cytoskeletal element distinct from any NF subunit, colocalized with phosphorylated NF-H immunoreactivity in many dystrophic elements in aged sympathetic prevertebral ganglia, a result which suggests a shared defect in a degradative mechanism or the accumulation of a possible hybrid filament. Recent work on cytoskeletal changes in diabetic somatic sensory neuropathy have identified a similar hyperphosphorylation of NF protein, thought to reflect increased activity of several MAP kinases [43].

The Autonomic Nervous System of Aged Experimental Animals

A variety of animal models have been developed in an attempt to determine the pathogenetic mechanisms underlying age-related autonomic neuropathy.

Pathophysiological and Biochemical Studies
Heart rate and arterial blood pressure are abnormal in aged rats [44], a finding thought to reflect age-related degeneration of cardiac noradrenergic innervation [45], altered norepinephrine turnover [46], or loss of functioning Ca^{2+} channels [47]. Thermoregulative abnormalities are a function of increased sympathetic nerve traffic to brown fat in the presence of defective postreceptor signal transduction [48]. Increased colonic transit time [48] in aged rats may reflect dysfunction of local reflexes underlying effective peristaltic activity, which are dependent on connections integrated in sympathetic prevertebral ganglia. Abnormal bladder function in aged rats may reflect reduced afferent input [49]. The sympathetic response of aged rats to a variety of experimental stressors (e.g., reserpine, fasting, heating, immobilization stress) may reveal pathology not present at their unstressed baseline [50–56].

Norepinephrine content (a coarse measure of sympathetic ganglionic health) has been reported to be decreased in aged rat CG, SMG and hypogastric ganglia [57, 58], although the activities of catecholamine synthetic enzymes

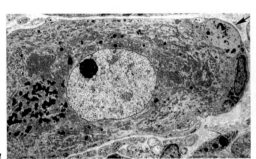
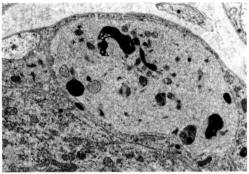

Fig. 3. Neuroaxonal dystrophy in aged rat SMG. A dystrophic axon (arrow, *a*) containing a variety of subcellular organelles (seen at higher magnification in 2*b*) is adjacent to a principal sympathetic neuron and enveloped in a satellite cell process. *a* 4,310×; *b* 18,210×.

TH and DβH are not decreased [54, 59]. Choline acetyltransferase, an enzyme marker predominantly located in presynaptic cholinergic elements, is variously reported as unchanged or increased in aged rat SCG [54, 59]. Decreased activity of succinate dehydrogenase [60], an important enzyme involved in oxidative phosphorylation, has been reported in aged rat SCG and CG/SMG and may represent increased glycolytic pathway activity intended to compensate for decreased oxidative metabolism; however, more recent studies have not found an expected change in baseline cytochrome oxidase activity [61].

The sympathetic nervous system does not operate in a vacuum and its alteration may interplay with the age-related changes in the parasympathetic nervous system (e.g., cardiac-vagal chemoreflex hyperresponse and baroreflex hypofunction [62]) which is understudied in aged experimental animals.

Neuropathology

The pathologic alterations of aged rat neurons of the sympathetic intermediolateral column prominently involved their dendritic structure [63, 64] rather than neuron loss. The neuronal complement of the sympathetic ganglia and hypogastric ganglia (a mixed sympathetic and parasympathetic ganglion) of aged rodents is well preserved [65–69] as is the preganglionic trunk to the SCG [70], evidence of preservation of the preganglionic sympathetic neurons.

As in humans, NAD represents a consistent hallmark of the aged sympathetic nervous system in rats [71] (fig. 3a, b), Chinese hamsters [72], and mice [73, 74]. Sympathetic ganglia of aged rodents are valid models of aging in human sympathetic ganglia. Both aged rodents and man: (1) develop NAD, but not substantive neuron loss, involving preterminal axons and synapses in aged sympathetic ganglia; (2) demonstrate a selectivity of NAD for prevertebral SMG and CG relative to paravertebral SCG and stellate ganglia; (3) develop neuropathologic changes ultrastructurally, immunohistochemically and anatomically identical to those in diabetics, and (4) demonstrate a predilection for NAD to target some subpopulations of nerve terminals while completely sparing others. In addition to NAD, there also may be concomitant alterations in the numbers of normal intraganglionic nerve terminals [75], either increased or decreased numbers, admixed with NAD. The dendritic arborization of intracellularly labeled CG/SMG neurons of young adult mice was significantly more complex and extensive than that of the SCG, and aged animals showed a relatively well-preserved CG/SMG dendritic apparatus [73]. Aged mouse SCG neurons, however, appeared significantly smaller with regard to total dendritic length and branching, in comparison to those of young animals, and exhibited short, stunted dendritic processes, results which have also been reported in aged rat SCG [76]. Studies of the aged rat hypogastric ganglion, which is composed of an unusual admixture of sympathetic and parasympathetic neuronal cell bodies, showed decreased numbers of synapsin-immunoreactive nerve terminals in relation to individual sympathetic neurons but normal numbers of nerve endings on parasympathetic neurons [75]. A detailed study of the sympathetic/parasympathetic composite major pelvic ganglion and preganglionic elements in aged male rats similarly identified reduction in the number of sympathetic preganglionic neurons, alterations in their dendritic structure and complexity, and reduced glutaminergic (but not glycinergic or GABA-immunoreactive) synaptic contact nerve endings on sympathetic preganglionic neurons but not on parasympathetic preganglionic neurons [77]. Serotonin- and TRH-immunoreactive nerve terminals were decreased on sympathetic preganglionic neurons innervating aged rat major pelvic ganglion but not on parasympathetic spinal nuclei [77].

Recent studies in aged mice [73, 74] have demonstrated a novel, pathologically distinct, marked dilatation of neurites (involving mostly axons but including dendrites as well) by numerous vacuoles which has been designated 'vacuolar neuritic dystrophy' (VND) and is essentially confined to the aged mouse SCG. Although the cervical sympathetic trunk (the preganglionic projection to the SCG) distant from the SCG never contained VND lesions, the majority of VND lesions in the aged SCG were lost following surgical interruption of the cervical sympathetic trunk, a result which is consistent with a distal process directed selectively against terminal axons and synapses. Intraneuronal injection experiments also demonstrated loss of dendritic arborization and focal dendritic swellings in the aged mouse SCG [73]. Sequential sectioning of ganglia and ultrastructural demonstration of dendritic characteristics of some dystrophic elements, suggested that VND in aged mouse SCG was not confined to axons and presynaptic elements. Rarely, VND arose from principal dendrites or from aberrant spine-like processes directly from the neuronal perikarya. VND was 30- to 100-fold more frequent in the aged mouse paravertebral SCG than in the prevertebral CG/SMG sympathetic ganglia of the same animals, again suggesting that the response of the sympathetic nervous system to age-related insults is heterogeneous. Sequential sections of aged ganglia heavily involved by VND demonstrated that most principal sympathetic neurons were contacted at some point by NAD, that the majority of dystrophic lesions arose from preterminal axons of essentially normal caliber and that multiple dystrophic elements often arose from a single axon and surrounded individual neurons as a basket. The ultrastructural appearance of individual VND lesions was identical in young and aged mice, differing only in frequency. Surprisingly, the frequency of VND in 22- to 27-month-old NIA-supplied mice was strain dependent, varying as much as 30-fold between DBA and C57BL6 strains, which represent the most and least VND-involved strains, respectively. VND exhibited a prominent gender effect (males had 3-fold more severe VND than females of a comparable age). Caloric restriction in mice, which significantly extends lifespan, presumably as a function of decreased oxidative stress, resulted in 70% fewer VND lesions than in age- and sex-matched controls fed ad libitum [74].

In addition to dystrophic alterations involving axon terminals contacting prevertebral principal sympathetic neurons, investigators have also reported an apparent decrease in distal postganglionic sympathetic noradrenergic axons and nerve terminals in a variety of target tissues including the rat heart, middle cerebral artery, ileum, kidney, bladder, pineal gland, spleen, mystacial pad and the cholinergic sympathetic innervation of sweat glands but not the iris or submandibular gland [45, 65, 78–86]. Interestingly, the loss of norepinephrine and serotonin innervation of aged guinea pig vasculature was accompanied by an increase in the vasodilator neurotransmitters VIP and CGRP [87], suggesting that attempting to correlate functional consequences of the loss of populations of sympathetic axons in isolation may be problematic. A recent study of age-related alterations in the innervation of gastrointestinal sphincters shows an increase in the density of excitatory neurotransmitters norepinephrine and substance P as well as a decreased density of inhibitory substances VIP and CGRP [88]. Other studies of aged rats demonstrated dendritic atrophy of the SCG neurons innervating the middle cerebral artery – which was reversed by local application of NGF [89] –, but not of those neurons innervating the iris [90]. A similar pattern of decreased NF gene expression has also been demonstrated for SCG neurons projecting to the middle cerebral artery but not those distributed to the iris [90]. There is, therefore, no compelling evidence that sympathetic autonomic aging in rats is uniform, resulting in a global loss of peripheral sympathetic endorgan innervation.

Alimentary dysfunction in aged rats may also reflect loss of enteric neurons [91], which may vary in degree from one level of the gut to another [92]. In addition, multiple subpopulations of enteric neurons may be differentially targeted by the aging process. In aged rats, significant loss in calbindin-immunoreactive neurons, which may represent intrinsic neurons with a sensory function, contrasts with the relative preservation of serotonin-immunoreactive myenteric neurons [93].

Postulated Mechanisms of Autonomic Nervous System Damage with Age

There is little evidence for the wholesale loss of significant numbers of neurons in aged autonomic ganglia. Instead, reproducible significant ganglionic pathology involves dendritic alterations, changes in synapse number or structure and NAD. Ganglionic pathology may be further complicated by the superimposition of significant losses of postganglionic sympathetic axonal projections or synapse-selective processes, which may vary from one endorgan to another.

Although NAD is characteristic of age-related changes in sympathetic ganglia, its distinctive pathology is not confined to aged sympathetic ganglia, and may be found in a variety of other age-related (gracile nucleus), toxic (bromophenylacetylurea, zinc pyridinethione intoxications), degenerative (Alzheimer's disease), genetic (infantile neuroaxonal dystrophy, Hallervorden-Spatz disease), metabolic (vitamin E deficiency) and neurotraumatic disorders involving the central and peripheral nervous system of man and experimental animals [94]. Mechanisms relevant to the pathogenesis of NAD in the relatively simple aging peripheral nervous system may be extrapolated to a variety of more complex disease processes in the central nervous system.

The mechanisms underlying age-related damage to the peripheral nervous system remain largely unknown; however, several hypotheses have been advanced [32].

Oxidative Injury
Oxidative stress results from a variety of physiologic and pathophysiologic pathways (e.g., mitochondrial function, catecholamine metabolism, ischemia, formation of glycated proteins) that may generate increased amounts of reactive oxygen species in aged animals, particularly in nerve terminals. Coupled with a reduction in antioxidant defenses (e.g., decreased levels of reduced glutathione, glutathione peroxidase and superoxide dismutase activities) increased amounts of reactive oxygen species are thought to contribute to a variety of age-related insults to the nervous system. Experimental lipid peroxidation of rat brain

synaptosomes results in alterations in membrane fluidity, lipid composition and Na^+-K^+ATPase activity, similar to changes produced by aging itself, which result in greater susceptibility of aged synaptic membranes to additional in vitro lipid peroxidation [95]. Oxidative stress may directly damage the mitochondrial genome resulting in dysfunctional mitochondria that produce increased amounts of free radicals which leak into the surrounding cytoplasm or produce further mitochondrial damage [4, 96, 97]. In support of this, reactive oxygen species have been reported to produce oxidized proteins which accumulate in synaptic mitochondria in old mice [98]. Increased indices of oxidative stress (tissue levels of malondialdehyde, 4-hydroxynonenal (4-HNE), protein carbonyls and decreased levels of GSH) have also been reported in the diabetic rat peripheral nervous system [99] which develops ganglionic pathology similar to that in aged ganglia. In a normal state, superoxide is degraded by superoxide dismutase; however, if the amount of superoxide produced overwhelms this capacity, super-oxide is converted to hydroxyl radical, a potent oxidant which targets a variety of intracellular macromolecules, chief among them polyunsaturated fatty acids resulting in the generation of 4-hydroxynonenal (4-HNE) [100, 101]. 4-HNE binds to several amino acids in a variety of intracellular proteins, interfering with their function. In addition, treatment of cultures with 4-HNE has been reported to interfere with the function of proteosomes, nonlysosomal cytosomes that function in the degradation of abnormal proteins [102], which may represent a link between oxidative damage and accumulation of intra-axonal organelles that represents a conspicuous characteristic of NAD.

Oxidative stress is closely associated with the development of NAD in several clinical and experimental conditions. Deficiency of the antioxidant vitamin E results in the premature and exaggerated development of NAD in aged human and rat primary sensory axon medullary terminals [103], which is sensitive to antioxidants and free radical scavengers. Studies in diabetic rats, which develop NAD identical in ganglionic distribution and ultrastructural appearance to that in aged rats, have provided additional support for oxidative stress in the pathogenesis and treatment of diabetic neuropathy. Recent studies [104] of diabetic autonomic neuropathy in rats have demonstrated that inhibitors of selected portions of the polyol pathway result in substantially decreased NAD (aldose reductase inhibitors) or significant worsening of NAD (sorbitol dehydrogenase inhibitors), a result which parallels the known effect of these agents to diminish or increase, respectively, markers of oxidative stress [105, 106]. Restriction of caloric intake (known to decrease oxidative damage in rodents) [107], significantly decreases dystrophic synaptic pathology in aged mouse SCG [74]. We have shown that increased sympathetic NAD in diabetic rats is nearly eliminated by IGF-I treatment in doses too small to significantly affect blood glucose levels [108], a result consistent with, although not limited to, the antioxidant effect of IGF-I. IGF-I has also been reported to protect dorsal root ganglion neurons from glucose-induced injury, a mechanism also known to involve oxidative stress [109].

Deficiency of Neurotrophic Substances and Aging in the Peripheral Nervous System

It has been proposed that the trophic support of endorgans on their innervating neurons may decline in old age due to decreased availability of target-derived neurotrophic substances [110–114] or alterations in receptor expression. Transplantation of aged or young endorgan targets into the anterior eye chamber of aged or young rats has demonstrated both target [109, 115]- and neuron-derived defects [116]. Other studies have reported deficient sympathetic sprouting into aged hippocampus [117] or sweat glands [115]. Exogenous treatment with NGF increased the sympathetic innervation density on both young and old targets, although not to the same degree [116, 118]. SCG neurons giving rise to the noradrenergic innervation of the middle cerebral artery, which decreases its total innervation by half with age, are reported to show NGF-reversible dendritic atrophy [119] in the absence of a decrease in NGF protein levels in the circle of Willis [120]. NGF content of blood vessels, pineal gland, submandibular glands and iris is not generally reduced in aged animals and age-related changes in endorgan nerve density do not correlate accurately with endorgan NGF content [114, 115, 120, 121]. Reinnervation of transplanted blood vessels by aged neurons is increased by exogenously administered NGF, but to a lesser extent than with young host neurons [116], which may reflect age-related decreased neuronal plasticity. The aged sympathetic nervous system may show an impaired response to low doses of NGF [114], although other studies suggest little decline in the capability of aged neurons to respond to intraventricular NGF [122]. Exposure of sympathetic neurons to anti-NGF is reported to produce atrophy of aged but not mature neurons, suggesting a decreased ability to scavenge NGF with age [123]. Decreased levels of p75^{NTR} (the low-affinity neurotrophin receptor) as well as mRNA for p75^{NTR} and trkA, the high-affinity receptor responding primarily to NGF [112, 124] have been reported in aged sympathetic ganglia. Other studies of aged rats have demonstrated dendritic atrophy and decreased NF gene expression of the SCG neurons innervating the middle cerebral artery (reversed by local application of NGF) [89], but not of those neurons innervating the iris [89, 90]. Neurons which innervate blood vessels are smaller and exhibit lower levels of NGF uptake (which declines with age) in contrast to iris-projecting neurons which are larger and take up greater amounts of NGF (a process which does not decline with age) [125].

Some of the apparent discrepancies between experiments identifying a target- or endorgan-derived defect in aged animals may reflect the differences between impaired collateral reinnervation in old animals [116], a process which is neurotrophin sensitive [126], and the retained capacity for axonal regeneration in aged rats [127], a neurotrophin-insensitive process [111, 128]. Animals with deficiency of sensory collateral sprouting (but not axonal regeneration), result from the administration of a course of anti-NGF into neonatal rats or by targeted disruption of p75^{NTR} in mice [129]. Septal lesion-induced collateral sprouting of sympathetic axons into the aged rat hippocampus is also reduced in the presence of diminished hippocampal NGF upregulation [113, 130]. A physiologic defect in sprouting of uninjured noradrenergic fibers within the pineal gland following extirpation of one SCG has been reported in aged in comparison to young rats [131]. Cycles of synaptic degeneration and regeneration may have more in common with collateral sprouting than long distance regeneration in terms of neurotrophin sensitivity, particularly if turnover involves replacement of degenerated terminals with adjacent axonal sprouts. Synaptic maintenance, plasticity, turnover, and collateral sprouting of axons may make use of shared basic processes which are differentially sensitive to a variety of neurotrophic substances.

Insulin and the insulin-like growth factors support the development and growth of sympathetic neurons in culture [132]. Insulin-like growth factor I (IGF-I) is thought to contribute to synaptic development, axonal sprouting and regeneration [133–136]. Administration of exogenous IGF-I to diabetic rats with established NAD in the SMG resulted in nearly complete reversal of NAD after 2 months [108] in the absence of a salutary effect on the severity of diabetes. The injury-induced increase in IGF-I content in the distal stump of axotomized sciatic nerve is reportedly blunted in aging [137]. IGF-I deficiencies identified in both aging and diabetes [138, 139] could contribute to abnormal synaptic turnover and the development of ganglionic NAD in both conditions. Significantly, IGF-I is also known to protect DRG neurons against oxidative insult by reactive oxygen species in vitro [109]. However, recent work [reviewed in ref. 140] has suggested that the relationship of aging insults to decreased signaling by IGFs may be more complex since reduced signaling by insulin-like peptides has been shown to increase the life span of a number of experimental species.

Neurotrophic Substances in Excess as a Pathogenetic
Mechanism for NAD

Alternatively, excessive amounts of neurotrophic substances may induce uncontrolled neuritic growth. This mechanism has been suggested to explain the neuritic swellings and apparent axonal sprouts in senile plaques of Alzheimer's disease which are rich in fibroblast growth factor (FGF) [141]. Neonatal sympathetic ganglia treated with 6-hydroxydopamine and high doses of NGF in vivo

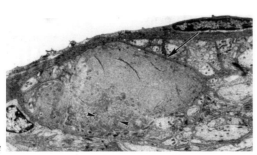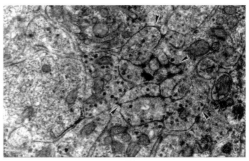

Fig. 4. Association of NAD and regenerative axonal sprouts in aged rat SMG. A massively swollen dystrophic axon (arrow, *a*) is associated with regenerative axonal sprouts (arrowheads, *a*), seen better at higher magnification in 3*b* (arrowheads). These delicate (0.1–0.2 μm) structures, similar those which originate from an axotomized parent axon in peripheral nerve regeneration, presumably subserve a similar function within sympathetic ganglia, although perhaps without the orientation supplied by Schwann cell tubes of regenerating peripheral nerve axons. *a* 4,950×; *b* 32,420×.

develop large intraganglionic swellings containing a variety of subcellular organelles which are reminiscent of NAD and suggest a pathogenetic role for coupled peripheral injury and increased ganglionic NGF [142]. Studies of autonomic neuropathy in diabetic rats have demonstrated that NAD identical to that found in aged rat ganglia develops prematurely and with increased severity in the diabetic prevertebral SMG and CG but not SCG [143]. Measurement of endogenous ganglionic NGF by ELISA [144] showed a doubling of NGF content in the diabetic CG and SMG but no consistent effect in the SCG, a distribution which parallels the development of ganglionic NAD. Systemic administration of exogenous NGF to adult control rats for 3 months has been shown to produce a doubling of NAD in the SMG [145]. Axonopathy may interfere with the retrograde transport of neurotrophic substances further contributing to a local excess in endorgans and the development of a self-perpetuating cycle. Increased NGF and other neurotrophins have also been shown to potentiate free radical-mediated neuronal death in some experimental paradigms [146–148].

Regenerative Mechanisms (Axonal Regeneration, Collateral Axonal Sprouting, Synaptic Plasticity)

The ultrastructural resemblance of some dystrophic axons to growth cones [94], the terminal motile tips of developing and regenerating axons, the frequent association of NAD with regenerative axonal sprouts [149, 150] (fig. 4) and its induction by frustration of peripheral axonal regeneration [151] suggest a relationship of NAD to abnormal axonal regeneration/collateral sprouting.

Synaptic turnover, a continuous normal process which may represent the structural equivalent of synaptic remodeling or 'plasticity' [152, 153], may share
mechanisms with collateral sprouting (i.e., neurotrophin-sensitive sprouting of
uninjured axons into denervated targets) and axonal regeneration (neurotrophin-
insensitive regrowth of previously injured axons) [128]. Axonal regeneration
and, particularly, collateral sprouting are deficient in various organs of aged
animals [117, 126, 131, 154, 155]. Synaptic turnover in autonomic ganglia may
be further complicated in pathologic states by superimposed postganglionic
axotomy, which itself results in the detachment, swelling and retraction of
presynaptic elements, a process which may represent an exaggerated form of
normal synaptic turnover and may represent the substrate from which NAD
develops. Finally, regeneration of nerve terminals must eventually cease (i.e.,
initiate a 'stop' program) to reform a stable nerve terminal. The inhibition of the
stop program has been reported to result in swollen nerve terminals, reminiscent of NAD [156].

Synaptic Degradation of Organelles

NF undergo orthograde transport to the nerve terminal but are not returned
intact and, instead, undergo degradation by calcium-activated neutral proteases
(calpains). Postsynthetic modification of NF by glycosylation resulting in the
formation of advanced glycosylation endproducts [157, 158], a process which
is thought to operate in both aging and diabetes, or by excessive phosphorylation may change the sensitivity of NF to calpains and other proteases, which
could result in their excessive accumulation in axonal terminals.

Extracellular Matrix

Detailed studies [159] of the normal process of removal of supernumerary
neuromuscular junctions suggest a seminal role for alterations in the matrix and
postsynaptic elements in the loss of presynaptic nerve terminals. Neural cell
adhesion molecule (NCAM) may promote or inhibit synaptic plasticity or
stability as the result of alternative splicing or postranslational polysialation
[160]. Cultured aged SCG neurons exhibit diminished responsiveness to laminin
in the presence of NGF [161, 162] and reduced laminin immunoreactivity is
reported to correlate with decreased innervation (possibly due to a defect in
collateral sprouting) of middle cerebral artery walls of aging rats in vivo [163,
164]. Age-related alterations in the extracellular matrix are, thus, also capable of
affecting nerve terminal structure, function and plasticity. Conversely, sympathetic neurons cultured on an aged or young central nervous system frozen
section substrate (an environment with extracellular matrix and possible bound
neurotrophic substances) show region-specific but not age-related differences [165].

Abnormal Calcium Dynamics

Norepinephrine release and abnormal calcium handling by aged SCG neurons in culture and the noradrenergic innervation of the aged rat tail vasculature are thought to reflect an age-related decline in Ca^{2+} uptake by smooth endoplasmic reticulum and increased reliance on mitochondrial calcium buffering [166, 167]. A decline in Ca^{2+}ATPase activity in the smooth endo-plasmic reticulum of aged rat SCG neurons may result in increased stimulation-evoked release of norepinephrine in older adrenergic nerves [168]. Several recent studies of aged rat sympathetic pelvic ganglion neurons show a decrease in calbindin and neurocalcin immunoreactivity, alterations which may also contribute to impaired intracellular Ca^{2+} buffering and Ca^{2+}-dependent signaling [169, 170]. The precise control of intracellular Ca^{2+} concentration is important for a variety of critical cellular processes including degradative calpain-mediated cytoskeletal turnover.

In summary, age-related sympathetic dysfunction is not thought to result from a generalized and progressive loss of neurons in human sympathetic ganglia; rather, alterations in the number, subtype and structure of presynaptic elements are poised to interfere with integration of visceral reflexes. Comparable damage to the distalmost portions of the postganglionic sympa-thetic innervation of endorgans may further amplify the dysfunction wrought by intraganglionic pathology, although quantitative studies of age-related dam-age to sympathetic endorgan innervation are rare. Recent studies of the sympa-thetic nervous system of human subjects and development of valid animal models have contributed to our understanding of the pathogenesis and possible treatment of autonomic dysfunction in aging. Pathologic processes targeting the synapse interrupt the most precarious site for neuronal transmission of the nerve impulse and may have significant consequences far more substantial than a modest degree of neuron loss, particularly for integrated nervous functions. Aging may selectively target plasticity-related synaptic remodeling. Abnormalities of synaptic turnover, therefore, may affect the most complex and critical processes in the peripheral and central nervous systems. Studies of the pathogenesis of NAD and synaptic dysplasia in the relatively simple peripheral nervous system may provide more general insight into the mechanisms which underlie more complex CNS processes (e.g., neurotrauma, neurodegenerative and inherited diseases) in which similarities in pathology may reflect shared mechanisms. NAD, synaptic loss and dendritic alterations are the neuropatho-logic hallmarks of aging in the human and rodent sympathetic nervous system. Although dystrophic changes in intraganglionic terminal axons and synapses are a robust, unequivocal and consistent neuropathologic finding in the aged sympathetic nervous system of man and animals, they may only represent the most visible residua of a more insidious synapse-directed process. The fidelity of animal models to the neuropathology of aged humans suggests that similar pathogenic mechanisms may be involved in both and that therapeutic advances in animal studies may presage human application.

Acknowledgements

The work from the author's laboratory has been supported by NIH grants AG10299 and DK19645. The author would like to thank Angela Schmeckebier for help with figure 1.

References

1 Schmidt RE: The aging autonomic nervous system; in Duckett S, de La Torre J (eds): Pathology of the Aging Human Nervous System. Oxford, Oxford University Press, 2001, pp 527–545.
2 Amenta F: Aging of the Autonomic Nervous System. Boca Raton, CRC Press, 1993.
3 Lipsitz LA: Aging and the autonomic nervous system; in Robertson D, Low PA, Polinsky RJ (eds): Primer on the Autonomic Nervous System. San Diego, Academic Press, 1996, pp 79–83.
4 Low PA: The effect of aging on the autonomic nervous system; in Low PA (ed): Clinical Autonomic Disorders. Evaluation and Management. Philadelphia, Lippincott-Raven, 1997, pp 161–175.
5 Catz A, Korczyn AD: Aging and the autonomic nervous system; in Appenzeller O (ed): Handbook of Clinical Neurology. Amsterdam, Elsevier, vol 74, 1999, pp 225–243.
6 Collins KF, Dore C, Exton-Smith AN, Fox RH, MacDonald IC, Woodward PM: Accidental hypothermia and impaired temperature homeostasis in the elderly. Br Med J 1977;i:353–356.
7 Geboes K, Bossaert H: Gastrointestinal disorders in old age. Age Aging 1977;6:197–200.
8 Anuras S, Leoning-Baucke V: Gastrointestinal motility in the elderly. J Am Geriatr Soc 1984;32:386–398.
9 Anuras S, Sutherland J: Small intestinal manometry in healthy elderly subjects. J Am Geriatr Soc 1984;32:581–583.
10 Pfeifer MA, Weinberg CR, Cook D, Best JD, Reenan A, Halter JB: Differential changes of autonomic nervous system function with age in man. Am J Med 1983;75:249–258.
11 Bitsios P, Prettyman R, Szabadi E: Changes in autonomic function with age: A study of pupillary kinetics in healthy young and old people. Age Aging 1996;25:432–438.
12 Caird FI, Andrews GR, Kennedy RD: Effect of posture on blood pressure in the elderly. Br Heart J 1973;35:527–530.
13 Piccirillo G, Bucca C, Bauco C, Cinti AM, Michelle D, Fimognari FL, Cacciafixta M, Marigliano V: Power spectral analysis of heart rate in subjects over a hundred years old. Int J Cardiol 1998;63:53–61.
14 Ziegler D, Laux G, Dannehl K, Spuler M, Muhlen H, Mayer P, Gries FA: Assessment of cardiovascular autonomic function: Age-related normal ranges and reproducibility of spectral analysis, vector analysis, and standard tests of heart rate variation and blood pressure responses. Diabetic Med 1992;9:166–175.
15 Dillon N, Chung S, Kelly J, O'Malley K: Age and beta adrenoceptor-mediated function. Clin Pharmacol Ther 1980;27:769–772.
16 Lakatta EG: Cardiovascular regulatory mechanisms in advanced age. Physiol Rev 1993;73:413–467.
17 White M, Roden R, Minobe W, Khan MF, Larrabee P, Wollmering M, Post JD, Anderson F, Campbell D, Feldman D: Age-related changes in β-adrenergic neuroeffector systems in the human heart. Circulation 1994;90:1225–1238.
18 Docherty JR: Cardiovascular responses in aging. Pharmacol Rev 1990;42:103–125.
19 Roth GS, Joseph JA, Mason RP: Membrane alterations as causes of impaired signal transduction in Alzheimer's disease and aging. Trends Neurosci 1995;18:203–206.

20   Iwase S, Mano T, Watanabe T, Saito M, Kobayashi F: Age-related changes of sympathetic outflow to muscles in humans. J Gerontol 1990;46:M1–M5.
21   Ng AV, Callister R, Johnson DG, Seals DR: Sympathetic neural reactivity to stress does not increase with age in healthy humans. Am J Physiol 1994;267:H344–H353.
22   Palmer GJ, Ziegler MG, Lake CR: Response of norepinephrine and blood pressure to stress increases with age. J Gerontol 1978;33:482–487.
23   Rowe JW, Troen BR: Sympathetic nervous system and aging in man. Endocr Rev 1980;1:167–179.
24   Kreulen DL: Integration in autonomic ganglia. Physiologist 1984;27:49–55.
25   Schmidt RE, Chae HY, Parvin CA, Roth KA: Neuroaxonal dystrophy in aging human sympathetic ganglia. Am J Pathol 1990;136:327–338.
26   Schmidt RE, Plurad SB, Parvin CA, Roth KA: Effect of diabetes and aging on human sympathetic autonomic ganglia. Am J Pathol 1993;143:143–153.
27   Schmidt RE: Neuropathology of human sympathetic autonomic ganglia. Microsc Res Tech 1996; 35:107–121.
28   Dyck PJ, Jedrzejowska H, Karnes J, Kawamura Y, Low PA, O'Brien PC, Offord K, Ohnishi A, Ohta M, Pollock M, Stevens JC: Reconstruction of motor, sensory and autonomic neurons based on morphometric study of sampled levels. Muscle Nerve 1979;2:399–405.
29   Jarvi R, Helen P, Pelto-Huikko M, Rapoport SI, Hervonen A: Age-related changes on enkepha-linergic innervation of human sympathetic neurons. Mech Age Dev 1988;44:143–151.
30   Scaravilli F: Changes in neuronal structure and cell populations with ageing; in Thomas PK (ed): Peripheral Nerve Changes in the Elderly. New Issues in Neurosciences. Amsterdam, Wiley, 1988, vol 1, pp 95–107.
31   Kawasaki H, Murayama S, Tomonaga M, Izumiyama N, Shimada H: Neurofibrillary-tangles in human upper cervical ganglia. Morphological study with immunohistochemistry and electron microscopy. Acta Neuropathol 1987;75:156–159.
32   Schmidt RE: Synaptic dysplasia in sympathetic autonomic ganglia. J Neurocytol 1996;25:777–791.
33   Kuntz A: Histological variation in autonomic ganglia and ganglion cells associated with age and disease. Am J Pathol 1938;14:783–795.
34   Helen P, Zeitlin R, Hervonen A: Mitochondrial accumulations in nerve fibers of human sympa-thetic ganglia. Cell Tissue Res 1980;207:491–498.
35   Helen P: Fine-structural and degenerative features in adult and aged human sympathetic ganglion cells. Mech Aging Dev 1983;23:161–175.
36   Hervonen A: Age related neuropathologic changes in human sympathetic ganglia. Soc Neurosci Abstr 1984;10:451.
37   Schroer JA, Plurad SB, Schmidt RE: Fine structure of presynaptic axonal terminals in sympathetic autonomic ganglia of aging and diabetic human subjects. Synapse 1992;12:1–13.
38   Schmidt RE: Age-related sympathetic ganglionic neuropathology. Human pathology and animal models. Auton Neurosci 2002;96:63–72.
39   Schmidt RE, Dorsey DA, Roth KA: Immunohistochemical characterization of NPY and sub-stance P containing nerve terminals in aged and diabetic human sympathetic ganglia. Brain Res 1992;583:320–326.
40   Rios R, Stolfi A, Campbell PH, Pickoff AS: Postnatal development of the putative neuropeptide-Y-mediated sympathetic-parasympathetic autonomic interaction. Cardiovasc Res 1996;31:E96–E103.
41   Low PA, Okazaki H, Dyck PJ: Splanchnic preganglionic neurons in man. I. Morphometry of preganglionic cytons. Acta Neuropathol 1977;40:55–61.
42   Schmidt RE, Beaudet LN, Plurad SB, Dorsey DA: Axonal cytoskeletal pathology in aged and diabetic human sympathetic autonomic ganglia. Brain Res 1997;769:375–383.
43   Tomlinson DR: Mitogen-activated protein kinases as glucose transducers for diabetic complica-tions. Diabetologia 1999;42:1271–1281.
44   Roberts J, Goldberg PB: Changes in basic cardiovascular activities during the lifetime of the rat. Exp Aging Res 1976;2:487–517.
45   Goldberg PB, Kreider MS, McLean MR, Roberts J: Effects of aging at the adrenergic cardiac neuroeffector junction. Fed Proc 1986;45:45–47.
46   Kregel KC: Influence of aging on tissue-specific noradrenergic activity at rest and during non-exertional heating in rats. J Appl Physiol 1994;76:1226.

47 Snyder DL, Johnson MD, Aloyo VJ, Eskin B, Roberts J: Age-related changes in cardiac norepi-nephrine release: Role of calcium movement. J Gerontol 1995;50:B358–B367.
48 Florez-Duquet M, McDonald RB: Cold-induced thermoregulation and biological aging. Physiol Rev 1988;78:339–358.
49 Chai TC, Andersson KE, Tuttle JB, Steers WD: Altered neural control of micturition in the aged F344 rat. Urol Res 2000;28:348–354.
50 McDougal JN, Miller MS, Burks TF: Age-related changes in colonic function in rats. Am J Physiol 1984;247:G542–G546.
51 Weiss B, Greenberg L, Cantor E: Age-related alterations in the development of adrenergic dener-vation supersensitivity. Fed Proc 1979;38:1915–1921.
52 McCarty R: Sympathetic-adrenal medullary and cardiovascular responses to acute cold stress in adult and aged rats. J Auton Nerv Syst 1985;12:15–22.
53 Chiueh CC, Nespor SM, Rapoport SI: Cardiovascular, sympathetic and adrenal cortical respon-siveness of aged Fischer-344 rats to stress. Neurobiol Aging 1980;1:157–163.
54 Partanen M, Waller SB, London ED, Hervonen A: Indices of neurotransmitter synthesis and release in aging sympathetic nervous system. Neurobiol Aging 1985;6:227–232.
55 Rapoport EB, Young JB, Landsberg L: Impact of age on basal and diet induced changes in sympathetic nervous system activity of Fischer rats. J Gerontol 1981;36:152–157.
56 Kenney MJ, Fels RJ: Sympathetic nerve regulation to heating is altered in senescent rats. Am J Physiol 2002;283:R513–R520.
57 Partanen M, Santer RM, Hervonen A: The effect of aging on the histochemically demonstrable catecholamines in the hypogastric (major pelvic) ganglion of the rat. Histochem J 1980;12:527–535.
58 Santer RM, Partanen M, Hervonen A: Glycoxylic acid fluorescence and ultrastructural studies of neurones in the coeliac-superior mesenteric ganglia of the aged rat. Cell Tissue Res 1980;211: 475–485.
59 Reis DJ, Ross RA, Joh TH: Changes in the activity and amounts of enzymes synthesizing cate-cholamines and acetylcholine in brain, adrenal medulla, and sympathetic ganglia of aged rat and mouse. Brain Res 1977;136:465–474.
60 Baker DM, Santer RM: Development of a quantitative histochemical method for determination of succinate dehydrogenase activity in autonomic neurons and its application to the study of aging in the autonomic nervous system. J Histochem Cytochem 1990;38:525–531.
61 Warburton AL, Santer RM: Stability of enzymatic indicators of metabolic and neuronal activity in postganglionic neurons supplying the urinary tract of aged rats. Histochem J 1998;30:317–324.
62 Franchini KG, Moreira ED, Ida F, Krieger EM: Alterations in the cardiovascular control by the chemoreflex and baroreflex in old rats. Am J Physiol 1996;270:R310.
63 Dering MA, Santer RM, Watson AHD: Age-related changes in the morphology of preganglionic neurons projecting to rat hypogastric ganglion. J Neurocytol 1996;25:555–563.
64 Dering MA, Santer RM, Watson AHD: Age-related changes in the morphology of preganglionic neurons projecting to the paracervical ganglion of nulliparous and multiparous rats. Brain Res 1998;780:245–252.
65 Santer RM: Sympathetic neuron numbers in ganglia of young and aged rats. J Auton Nerv Syst 1991;33:221–222.
66 Warburton AL, Santer RM: The hypogastric and thirteenth thoracic ganglia of the rat: Effects of age on the neurons and their extracellular environment. J Anat 1997;190:115–124.
67 Hervonen A, Partanen M, Helen P, Koistinaho J, Alho H, Baker DM, Johnson JE, Santer RM: The sympathetic neuron, a model of neuronal aging; in Panulea P, Paivarinta H, Soinila S (eds): Neurohistochemistry: Modern Methods and Applications. New York, Liss, 1986, pp 569–586.
68 Santer RM: Morphological evidence for the maintenance of the cervical sympathetic system in aged rats. Neurosci Lett 1991;130:248–250.
69 Cowen T: Ageing in the autonomic nervous system: A result of nerve target interactions. A review. Mech Age Dev 1993;68:163–173.
70 Santer RM: Quantitative analysis of the cervical sympathetic trunk in young adult and aged rats. Mech Age Dev 1993;67:289–298.
71 Schmidt RE, Plurad SB, Modert CW: Neuroaxonal dystrophy in the autonomic ganglia of aged rats. J Neuropathol Exp Neurol 1983;42:376–390.

72   Schmidt RE, Plurad DA, Plurad SB, Cogswell BE, Diani AR, Roth KA: Ultrastructural and immunohistochemical characterization of autonomic neuropathy in genetically diabetic Chinese hamsters. Lab Invest 1989;61:77–92.

73   Schmidt RE, Beaudet LN, Plurad SB, Snider WD, Ruit KG: Pathologic alterations in pre- and postsynaptic elements in aged mouse sympathetic ganglia. J Neurocytol 1995;24:189–206.

74   Schmidt RE, Dorsey DA, Beaudet LN, Plurad SB, Parvin CA, Bruch LA: Vacuolar neuritic dystrophy in aged mouse superior cervical sympathetic ganglia is strain-specific. Brain Res 1998;806:141–151.

75   Warburton AL, Santer RM: Decrease in synapsin I staining in the hypogastric ganglion of aged rats. Neurosci Lett 1995;194:157–160.

76   Andrews TJ, Li D, Halliwell J, Cowen T: The effect of age on dendrites in the rat superior cervical ganglion. J Anat 1994;184:111–117.

77   Santer RM, Dering MA, Ranson RN, Waboso HN, Watson AHD: Differential susceptibility to ageing of rat preganglionic neurons projecting to the major pelvic ganglion and of their afferent inputs. Auton Neurosci 2002;96:73–81.

78   Thrasivoulou C, Cowen T: Regulation of rat sympathetic nerve density by target tissues and NGF in maturity and old age. Eur J Neurosci 1995;7:381–387.

79   Baker DM, Santer RM: A quantitative study of the effects of age on the noradrenergic innervation of Auerbach's plexus in the rat. Mech Age Dev 1988;42:147–158.

80   Vega JA, Ricci A, Amenta F: Age-dependent changes of the sympathetic innervation of the rat kidney. Mech Age Dev 1990;54:185–196.

81   Warburton AL, Santer RM: Sympathetic and sensory innervation of the urinary tract in young adult and aged rats: A semi-quantitative histochemical and immunolocalization study. Histochem J 1994;26:127–133.

82   Kuchel GA: Alterations in target innervation and collateral sprouting in the aging sympathetic nervous system. Exp Neurol 1993;124:381–386.

83   Felten SY, Bellinger DL, Collier TJ, Coleman PD, Felten DL: Decreased sympathetic innervation of spleen in aged Fischer 344 rats. Neurobiol Aging 1987;8:159–165.

84   Fundin BT, Bergman E, Ulfhake B: Alterations in mystacial pad innervation in the aged rat. Exp Brain Res 1997;117:324–340.

85   Abdel-Rahman TA, Cowen T: Neurodegeneration in sweat glands and skin of aged rats. J Auton Nerv Syst 1993;46:55–63.

86   Andrews TJ, Cowen T: In vivo infusion of NGF induces the organotypic regrowth of perivascular nerves following their atrophy in aged rats. J Neurosci 1994;14:3048–3058.

87   Mione MC, Dhital KK, Amenta F, Burnstock G: An increase in the expression of neuropeptidergic vasodilator, but not vasoconstrictor, cerebrovascular nerves in aging rats. Brain Res 1988;460:103–113.

88   Belai A, Wheeler H, Burnstock G: Innervation of the rat gastrointestinal sphincters: Changes during development and ageing. Int J Dev Neurosci 1995;13:81–95.

89   Andrews TJ, Thrasivoulou C, Nesbit W, Cowen T: Target-specific differences in the dendritic morphology and neuropeptide content of neurons in the rat SCG during development and age. J Comp Neurol 1996;368:33–44.

90   Kuchel GA, Poon T, Irshad K, Richard C, Julien JP, Cowen T: Decreased neurofilament gene expression is an index of selective axonal hypotrophy in ageing. Neuroreport 1997;10:799–805.

91   Santer RM, Baker DM: Enteric neuron numbers and sizes in Auerbach's plexus in the small and large intestine of adult and aged rats. J Auton Nerv Syst 1988;25:59–67.

92   Phillips RJ, Powley TL: As the gut ages: Timetables for aging of innervation vary by organ in the Fischer 344 rat. J Comp Neurol 2001;434:358.

93   Wade PR: Aging and neural control of the GI tract I. Age-related changes in the enteric nervous system. Am J Physiol 2002;283:G489–G495.

94   Jellinger K: Neuroaxonal dystrophy: Its natural history and related disorders. Prog Neuropathol 1973;2:129–180.

95   Viani P, Cervato G, Fiorilli A, Cestaro B: Age-related differences in synaptosomal peroxidative damage and membrane properties. J Neurochem 1991;56:253–258.

96   Shigenaga MK, Hagen TM, Ames BN: Oxidative damage and mitochondrial decay in aging. Proc Natl Acad Sci USA 1994;91:10771–10778.

97   Wilson PD, Franks LM: The effect of age on mitochondrial ultrastructure and enzymes. Adv Exp Med Biol 1975;53:171–183.

98   Martinez M, Hernandez AI, Martinez N, Ferrandiz ML: Age-related increase in oxidized proteins in mouse synaptic mitochondria. Brain Res 1996;731:246–248.

99   Low PA, Kim KK, Tritschler HJ: The roles of oxidative stress and antioxidant treatment in experimental diabetic neuropathy. Diabetes 1997;46(suppl 2):S38–S42.

100 Smith LL: Paraquat toxicity. Phil Trans R Soc Lond B 1985;311:647–657.

101 Yang W, Sun AY: Paraquat-induced free radical reaction in mouse brain microsomes. Neurochem Res 1998;23:47–53.

102 Keller JN, Hanni KB, Markesbery WR: Possible involvement of proteosome inhibition in aging: Implications for oxidative stress. Mech Age Dev 2000;113:61–70.

103 Lampert PW, Blumberg JM, Pentshew A: An electron microscopic study of dystrophic axons in the gracile and cuneate nuclei of vitamin E deficient rats. J Neuropathol Exp Neurol 1964;23: 60–77.

104 Schmidt RE, Dorsey DA, Beaudet LN, Plurad SB, Williamson JR, Ido Y: Effect of sorbitol dehydrogenase inhibition on experimental diabetic autonomic neuropathy. J Neuropathol Exp Neurol 1998;57:1175–1189.

105 Obrosova IG, Fathallah L, Lang HJ, Greene DA: Evaluation of a sorbitol dehydrogenase inhibitor on diabetic peripheral nerve metabolism: A prevention study. Diabetologia 1999;42: 1187–1194.

106 Obrosova IG, Green DA, Lang HJ: Antioxidative defense in diabetic peripheral nerve: Effects of *DL*-α-lipoic acid, aldose reductase inhibitor, and sorbitol dehydrogenase inhibitor; in Packer L, Rösen P, Tritschler HJ, King GL, Azzi A (eds): Antioxidants in Diabetes Management. New York, Dekker, 1998, pp 93–110.

107 Sohal R, Weindruch R: Oxidative stress, caloric restriction and aging. Science 1996;273:59–63.

108 Schmidt RE, Dorsey DA, Beaudet LN, Plurad SB, Parvin CA, Miller MS: Insulin-like growth factor I reverses experimental diabetic autonomic neuropathy. Am J Pathol 1999;155:1651–1660.

109 Russell J, Golovoy D, Mahendru P, Feldman EL: IGF-I and inhibitors of oxidative stress block high glucose induced mitochondrial dysfunction and neuronal cell death. Soc Neurosci Abstr 2000;26:817.

110 Gavazzi I, Andrews TJ, Thrasivoulou C, Cowen T: Influence of target tissues on their innervation in old age: A transplantation study. Neuroreport 1992;3:717–720.

111 Gavazzi I, Cowen T: Can the neurotrophic hypothesis explain degeneration and loss of plasticity in mature and ageing autonomic nerves? J Auton Nerv Syst 1996;58:1–10.

112 Uchida Y, Tomonaga M: Loss of nerve growth factor receptors in sympathetic ganglia from aged mice. Biochem Biophys Res Commun 1987;146:797–801.

113 Scott SA, Liang S, Weingartner JA, Crutcher KA: Increased NGF-like activity in young but not aged rat hippocampus after septal lesions. Neurobiol Aging 1994;15:337–346.

114 Cowen T, Gavazzi I: Plasticity in adult and ageing sympathetic neurons. Prog Neurobiol 1998;54: 249–288.

115 Cowen T, Thrasivoulou C, Shaw SA, Abdel-Rahman TA: Transplanted sweat glands from mature and aged donors determine cholinergic phenotype an altered density of host sympathetic nerves. J Auton Nerv Syst 1996;58:153–162.

116 Gavazzi I: Collateral sprouting and responsiveness to nerve growth factor of ageing neurons. Neurosci Lett 1995;189:47–50.

117 Crutcher KA: Age-related decrease in sympathetic sprouting is primarily due to decreased target receptivity: Implications for understanding brain aging. Neurobiol Aging 1990;11:175–183.

118 Gavazzi I, Cowen T: NGF can induce a 'young' pattern of innervation in transplanted old cerebral blood vessels? J Comp Neurol 1993;334:489–496.

119 Andrews TJ, Cowen T: Nerve growth factor enhances the dendritic arborization of sympathetic ganglion cells undergoing atrophy in aged rats. J Neurocytol 1994;23:234–241.

120 Gavazzi I, Cowen T, Crutcher KA: Lack of correlation between NGF levels and altered nerve fibre density in peripheral tissues of aging rats. Soc Neurosci Abstr 1994;20:1710.

121 Kuchel GA, Crutcher KA, Naheed U, Thrasivoulou C, Cowen T: NGF expression in the aged rat pineal gland does not correlate with loss of sympathetic axonal branches and varicosities. Neurobiol Aging 1999;20:685–693.

122 Dickason AK, Isaacson LG: Plasticity of aged perivascular axons following exogenous NGF: Analysis of catechholamines. Neurobiol Aging 2002;23:125–134.

123 Gavazzi I, Canavan REM, Cowen T: Influence of age and anti-NGF treatment on the sympathetic and sensory innervation of the rat iris. Neuroscience 1996;73:1069–1079.

124 Kuchel GA, Rowe W, Meaney MJ, Richard C: Neurotrophin receptor and tyrosine hydroxylase gene expression in aged sympathetic neurons. Neurobiol Aging 1997;18:67–79.

125 Cowen T: Selective vulnerability in adult and ageing mammalian neurons. Auton Neurosci 2002; 96:20–24.

126 Gloster A, Diamond J: Sympathetic nerves in adult rats regenerate normally and restore pilomotor function during an anti-NGF treatment that prevents their collateral sprouting. J Comp Neurol 1992;326:363–374.

127 Gavazzi I, Cowen T: Axonal regeneration from transplanted sympathetic ganglia is not impaired by age. Exp Neurol 1993;122:57–64.

128 Mearow KM, Kril Y, Gloster A, Diamond J: Expression of NGF receptor and gap-43 mRNA in DRG neurons during collateral sprouting and regeneration of dorsal cutaneous nerves. J Neurobiol 1994;25:127–142.

129 Diamond J, Lourenssen S, Pertens E, Urschel B: Lack of collateral sprouting of nociceptive nerves in adult p75 knock-out mice. Soc Neurosci Abstr 1995;21:1539.

130 Milner TA, Loy R: Interaction of age and sex in sympathetic axon ingrowth into the hippocampus following septal afferent damage. Anat Embryol 1980;161:159–168.

131 Kuchel GA, Zigmond RE: Functional recovery and collateral neuronal sprouting examined in young and aged rats following a partial neural lesion. Brain Res 1991;540:195–203.

132 Recio-Pinto E, Rechler MM, Ishii DN: Effects of insulin, insulin-like growth factor-II, and nerve growth factor in neurite formation and survival in cultured sympathetic and sensory neurons. J Neurosci 1986;6:1211–1219.

133 Ishii DN, Glazner GW, Whalen LR: Regulation of peripheral nerve regeneration by insulin-like growth factors. Ann NY Acad Sci 1993;692:172–182.

134 Ishii DN, Glazner GW, Pu SF: Role of insulin-like growth factors in peripheral nerve regeneration. Pharmacol Ther 1994;62:125–144.

135 Cheng H-L, Randolph A, Yee D, Delafontaine P, Tennekoon G, Feldman EL: Characterization of insulin-like growth factor-I and its receptor and binding proteins in transected nerves and cultured Schwann cells. J Neurochem 1996;66:525–536.

136 Hansson H-A: Insulin-like growth factors and nerve regeneration. Ann NY Acad Sci 1993;692: 161–171.

137 D'Costa AP, Lenham JE, Ingram RL, Sonntag WE: Comparison of protein synthesis in brain and peripheral tissue during aging. Relationship to insulin-like growth factor-1 and type 1 IGF receptors. Ann NY Acad Sci 1993;692:253–255.

138 Tan K, Baxter RC: Serum insulin-like growth factor I levels in adult diabetic patients: The effect of age. J Clin Endocrinol Metab 1986;63:651–655.

139 Migdalis IN, Kalogeropoulou K, Kalantzis L, Nounopoulos C, Bouloukos A, Samartzis M: Insulin-like growth factor-I and IGF-I receptors in diabetic patients with neuropathy. Diabet Med 1995;12:823–827.

140 Tatar M, Bartke A, Antebi A: The endocrine regulation of aging by insulin-like signals. Science 2003;299:1346–1351.

141 Cotman CW, Gomez-Pinilla F: Basic fibroblast growth factor in the mature brain and its possible role in Alzheimer's disease. Ann NY Acad Sci 1991;638:221–231.

142 Levi-Montalcini R, Aloe L, Mugnaini E, Oesch F, Thoenen H: Nerve growth factor induces volume increase and enhances tyrosine hydroxylase synthesis in chemically axotomized sympathetic ganglia of newborn rats. Proc Natl Acad Sci USA 1975;72:595–599.

143 Schmidt RE, Plurad SB: Ultrastructural and biochemical characterization of autonomic neuropathy in rats with chronic streptozotocin diabetes. J Neuropathol Exp Neurol 1986;45: 525–544.

144 Schmidt RE, Dorsey DA, Roth KA, Parvin CA, Hounsom L, Tomlinson DR: Effect of streptozotocin-induced diabetes on NGF, p75[NTR] and Trk A content of prevertebral and paravertebral rat sympathetic ganglia. Brain Res, 2000;867:149–156.

145 Schmidt RE, Dorsey DA, Beaudet LN, Parvin CA, Escandon E: Effect of NGF and Neurotrophin-3 treatment on experimental diabetic autonomic neuropathy. J Neuropathol Exp Neurol 2001;60: 263–273.

146 Behrens MM, Strasser U, Lobner D, Dugan LL: Neurotrophin-mediated potentiation of neuronal injury. Microsc Res Tech 1999;45:276–284.

147 Pan Z, Perez-Polo R: Role of nerve growth factor in oxidant homeostasis: Glutathione metabolism. J Neurochem 1993;61:1713–1721.

148 McDonald JW, Stefovska VG, Liu XZ, Shin H, Liu S, Choi DW: Neurotrophin potentiation of iron-induced spinal cord injury. Neuroscience 2002;115:931–939.

149 Schmidt RE: Neuroaxonal dystrophy in aging rodent and human sympathetic autonomic ganglia: Synaptic pathology as a common theme in neuropathology. Adv Pathol Lab Med 1993; 6:505–522.

150 Schmidt RE, Scharp DW: Axonal dystrophy in experimental diabetic autonomic neuropathy. Diabetes 1982;31:761–770.

151 Ohara S, Beaudet LN, Schmidt RE: Transganglionic response of GAP-43 in the gracile nucleus to sciatic nerve injury in young and aged rats. Brain Res 1995;705:325–331.

152 Cotman CW, Nieto-Sampedro M, Harris EW: Synapse replacement in the nervous system of adult vertebrates. Physiol Rev 1981;61:684–784.

153 Purves D, Voyvodic JT, Magrassi L, Yawo H: Nerve terminal remodeling visualized in living mice by repeated examination of the same neurons. Science 1987;238:1122–1126.

154 Navarro X, Kennedy WR: Effect of age on collateral reinnervation of sweat glands in the mouse. Brain Res 1988;463:174–181.

155 Scheff SW, Bernardo LS, Cotman DW: Decrease in adrenergic axon sprouting in the senescent rat. Science 1978;202:775–778.

156 Liuzzi FJ: Proteolysis is a critical step in the physiological stop pathway: Mechanisms involved in the blockade of axonal regeneration by mammalian astrocytes. Brain Res 1990;512:277–283.

157 Vlassara H, Bucala R, Striker L: Pathogenic effects of advanced glycosylation: Biochemical, biologic, and clinical implications for diabetes and aging. Lab Invest 1994;70:138–151.

158 Yagihashi S, Kamijo M, Taniguchi N, Satoh K: Increased glycation of axonal cytoskeleton and preventive effect of aminoguanidine on development of experimental diabetic neuropathy. Diabetes 1991;40(suppl 1):302A.

159 Carbonetto S, Lindenbaum M: The basement membrane at the neuromuscular junction: A synaptic mediatrix. Curr Opin Neurobiol 1995;5:596–605.

160 Doherty P, Fazeli MS, Walsh FS: The neural cell adhesion molecule and synaptic plasticity. J Neurobiol 1995;26:437–446.

161 Jenner CS, Gavazzi I, Song GX, Cohen T: Loss of responsiveness of ageing sympathetic neurons in vitro to laminin and NGF. Eur J Neurosci 1994;7(suppl):185.

162 Cowen T, Jenner C, Xiao Song G, Santoso AW, Gavazzi I: Responses of mature and aged sympathetic neurons to laminin and NGF: An in vitro study. Neurochem Res 1997;22:1003–1011.

163 Gavazzi I, Boyle KS, Edgar D, Cowen T: Reduced laminin immunoreactivity in the blood vessel wall of ageing rats correlates with reduced innervation in vivo and following transplantation. Cell Tissue Res 1995;281:23–32.

164 Gavazzi I, Boyle KS, Cowen T: Extracellular matrix molecules influence innervation density in rat cerebral blood vessels. Brain Res 1996;734:167–174.

165 Pettigrew DB, Levin L, Crutcher KA: Sympathetic neurite growth on central nervous system sections is region-specific and unaltered by aging. Neurobiol Aging 2000;21:629–638.

166 Tsai H, Pottorf WJ, Buchholz JN, Duckles SP: Adrenergic nerve smooth endoplasmic reticulum calcium buffering declines with age. Neurobiol Aging 1998;89:89–96.

167 Toescu EC, Verkhratsky A: Parameters of calcium homeostasis in normal neuronal aging. J Anat 2000;197:563–569.

168 Tsai H, Pottorf WJ, Buchholz JN, Duckles SP: Adrenergic nerve smooth endoplasmic reticulum calcium buffering declines with age. Neurobiol Aging 1998;19:89–96.

169 Corns RA, Hidaka H, Santer RM: Decreased neurocalcin immunoreactivity in sympathetic and parasympathetic neurons of the major pelvic ganglion in aged rats. Neurosci Lett 2001;297:81–84.
170 Corns RA, Boolaky UV, Santer RM: Decreased calbindin-D28k immunoreactivity in aged rat sympathetic pelvic ganglionic neurons. Neurosci Lett 2000;292:91–94.

Robert E. Schmidt, MD, PhD
Department of Pathology and Immunology
Division of Neuropathology (Box 8118), Washington University School of Medicine
660 South Euclid Avenue, Saint Louis, MO 63110 (USA)
Tel. +1 314 362 7429, Fax +1 314 362 4096, E-Mail reschmidt@pathology.wustl.edu

Kuchel GA, Hof PR (eds): Autonomic Nervous System in Old Age.
Interdiscipl Top Gerontol. Basel, Karger, 2004, vol 33, pp 24–31

....

Clinical and Therapeutic Implications of Aging Changes in Autonomic Function

Gary A. Ford

Institute for Ageing and Health, University of Newcastle upon Tyne,
Newcastle upon Tyne, UK

Autonomic regulation of the involuntary functions of various organs and tissues is subject to significant changes in old age. Given the extensive changes that occur in the autonomic nervous system with aging and the physiological challenges faced by many older individuals, it is perhaps surprising how well the autonomic nervous system functions in maintaining the internal environment in the majority of older people.

Prescribing of drugs to older people has increased substantially in recent years due to changes in aging demographics. In the UK, older people now receive more than 50% all prescribed drug therapy, and this is likely to continue to increase, as increasing evidence of the benefits of drug treatment becomes available [1]. The response of older people to drug therapy is frequently altered due to both pharmacokinetic and pharmacodynamic changes [2]. Age-associated alterations in pharmacodynamics are less well described than pharmacokinetic changes in part because of the difficulties in studying pharmacodynamics. However, significant advances in understanding of age-associated alterations in pharmacodynamics have occurred in the last 25 years and many of these changes involve the autonomic nervous system.

This chapter will review the effect of aging changes in autonomic function on clinical problems and therapeutics in older people. Treatment of cardiovascular disorders will be the primary focus for discussion since these agents account for the largest proportion of prescribed drugs, and aging changes in the human cardiovascular autonomic nervous system have been well studied compared to other organ systems. The main age-associated changes in autonomic nervous system function and the clinical consequences are listed in table 1.

Table 1. Main age-associated changes in cardiovascular autonomic function and clinical consequences

Reduced β-adrenergic responsiveness
Reduced maximal heart rate, stroke volume and exercise capacity
Reduced bronchodilator response to inhaled β-agonists
Reduced awareness hypoglycemia
Increased SNS activity
Hypertension[1]
Decreased baroreflex sensitivity
Increased incidence orthostatic hypotension, vasovagal syndrome
Increased BP variability (as a consequence of baroreflex changes)
Increased incidence syncope and falls
Increased risk of cerebrovascular events[1]

[1]Causal association not proven.

Aging Changes in β-Adrenoceptor Responsiveness

The reduction in β-adrenoceptor responsiveness with age has been described in many but not all tissues. Although this finding was reported more than 30 years ago in humans, and confirmed in many animal models, there is still some controversy as to the extent of the reduction in cardiac β-adrenoceptor responsiveness that occurs with aging [3–5]. The consequences of this reduced responsiveness appear less than would be anticipated, perhaps because of the increase in sympathetic nervous system activity which provides a higher 'drive' to the receptors under both resting conditions and in situations where the sympathetic nervous system is activated. Indeed the age-associated reduction in β-adrenoceptor activity may be an adaptive response to the increased sympathetic nervous system activity. The age-associated reduction in maximal heart rate appears to be due to reduced cardiac chronotropic responsiveness of cardiac β-adrenoceptors to cardiac norepinephrine release during exercise [6]. The ability to increase cardiac output is more dependent on enhancing stroke volume, which is maintained in healthy older subjects due to an increase in left ventricular end diastolic volume. However, cardiac inotropic responsiveness is also reduced and the ability to increase cardiac output is diminished in many older subjects particularly when ischemic heart disease interacts with these age-associated changes.

The age-associated reduction in vascular β-adrenoceptor responsiveness can be modulated by salt restriction and exercise, which have both been reported to increase β-adrenoceptor responsiveness [7]. This effect may partially contribute to the blood pressure-lowering effects of these interventions in an older population. A causal association is supported by recent studies demonstrating correction of impaired β-adrenergic vasodilatation in hypertensive rats by $β_2$-adrenergic receptor gene delivery to the endothelium [8].

Reduced β-adrenoceptor responsiveness of bronchial smooth muscle would be expected to impair responsiveness of older individuals with obstructive pulmonary disease to inhaled $β_2$-adrenoceptor agonists, and a progressive age-associated reduction in response to inhaled β-adrenoceptor agonists has been reported [9]. In contrast, airway responsiveness to the antimuscarinic antagonist bronchodilators is unaffected by age.

Some evidence suggests that older subjects are less sensitive to β-adrenoceptor antagonists although comparing responses, such as falls in blood pressure between young and older patients, is methodologically problematic, and aging difference in responsiveness to β-blockers has been studied far less than in β-agonists [9]. There is no reason why diminished responsiveness to β-agonists would necessarily result in reduced responsiveness to β-blockers. However, the β-blocker atenolol is less effective than losartan in preventing stroke in middle- and older-aged hypertensives with left ventricular hypertrophy despite virtually identical falls in blood pressure [10]. Previous studies have also suggested β-blockers are less effective agents for prevention of stroke in treatment of hypertension [11].

A further consequence of the reduced β-adrenergic responsiveness is reduced awareness of older subjects of hypoglycemia. Although older subjects with diabetes mount a similar counter-regulatory hormone response to hypoglycemia they experience lower symptoms in response to this, due to reduced tachycardia and sweating in response to sympathetic nervous system activity. In contrast, cognitive deterioration when assessed by changes in visual reaction time and digit symbol substitution was similarly impaired in young and older subjects with diabetes experiencing hypoglycemia [12].

Aging Changes in Baroreflex Sensitivity

Reduced baroreflex sensitivity was one of the first alterations in autonomic function described with aging in humans and has important clinical implications [13, 14]. Reduced baroreflex sensitivity results in impaired ability of older people to maintain blood pressure within a narrow range, resulting in increased blood pressure variability and an increased likelihood of orthostatic hypotension. Other hypotensive disorders, such as vagovagal syncope and vasodepressor carotid sinus hypersensitivity are more common in the elderly, and also appear to be mediated through altered baroreflex sensitivity. Recent evidence indicates that aerobic exercise attenuates the age-associated decline in cardiac baroreflex sensitivity and can enhance sensitivity in previously sedentary middle-aged and older healthy men, which may account for benefits of aerobic exercise in lowering blood pressure [15, 16].

The reduction in baroreflex sensitivity leads to a greater likelihood of orthostatic hypotension in older people with blood pressure-lowering drugs [17]. Anecdotal evidence suggests this is especially problematic with α-adrenoceptor antagonists, particularly after the first dose because of the high prevalence of orthostatic hypotension with these agents [18]. Good comparative studies comparing prevalence of orthostatic hypotension with different classes of blood pressure-lowering agents in older people are lacking, although the angiotensin II receptor antagonists appear to be very well tolerated by older subjects with few withdrawals in clinical studies due to orthostatic hypotension [19].

The increase in blood pressure variability and failure of nocturnal dipping of blood pressure appear to be consequences of altered baroreflex function. Emerging evidence indicates that increased blood pressure variability is associated with an increased risk of myocardial infarction and stroke. Increased office diastolic blood pressure variability was higher in patients who had experienced myocardial infarction [20], and patients with lacunar cerebral infarcts due to small vessel disease were found to have a reduced nighttime fall in systolic blood pressure [21]. Prospective studies following the outcome of patients with increased blood pressure variability are needed to determine whether this relationship is causal. However both hypotension and hypertension could potentially precipitate cerebral infarction, particularly in small vessels. The ability to maintain systemic blood pressure and cerebral perfusion appears to be of key importance in protecting the older brain from cerebrovascular disease. Orthostatic hypotension was found to be an independent risk factor for stroke and coronary artery disease in a middle-aged population [22, 23]. In a small MRI study of 30 patients with orthostatic hypotension or carotid sinus hypersensitivity, the severity of MRI hyperintensities in deep white matter and basal ganglia was greater in patients with a blood pressure fall more than 30 mm Hg during provocation [24]. In a detailed study of hypertensive older subjects where magnetic resonance brain imaging studies were used to define cerebrovascular disease, orthostatic hypotension and orthostatic hypertension were both found to be associated with cerebrovascular disease [25]. Both orthostatic hypotension and orthostatic hypertension were associated with increased systolic blood pressure variability on ambulatory monitoring. Further work is needed to determine whether increased blood pressure variability is a cause or a consequence of cerebrovascular disease, although it seems likely that both mechanisms occur in older subjects. Clarifying the extent to which increased blood pressure variability is a cause of cerebrovascular disease would have important implications for optimal treatment of hypertension and hypotensive disorders in older people.

A key advance in clinical geriatrics has been the recognition that syncope and many falls in older people are frequently secondary to hypotensive disorders that arise secondary to autonomic dysfunction – a group of disorders including orthostatic hypotension, carotid sinus hypersensitivity, and vasovagal syndrome described as neurally mediated syncope [26–28]. Vasovagal syndrome and orthostatic hypotension are associated with reduced baroreflex sensitivity, which may account for their high prevalence in the older population [29]. Paradoxically, carotid sinus hypersensitivity, the other major cause of hypotension in older people is associated with increased baroreflex sensitivity, which is not consistent with the known blunting effects of aging on baroreflex sensitivity [30]. The cause of this increased sensitivity is unclear, but appears to be due to altered central responsiveness to nonphysiologic stimuli of the carotid sinus [31]. O'Mahony [30] has suggested a model in which upregulation of central α_2-adrenoceptors occurs secondary to reduced afferent impulse traffic to the baroreflex pathway. Such declines in afferent firing would, in turn, result from baroreflex postsynaptic hypersensitivity caused by reduced carotid sinus compliance due to hypertension and atherosclerosis [30]. As a result, stimulation of the carotid sinus could produce overshoot of efferent baroreflex responses with profound hypotension and bradycardia [30]. Further research is needed to understand the pathophysiology of hypotensive disorders in older people to inform the development of therapeutic interventions to improve blood pressure homeostasis in these patients.

Increased Sympathetic Nervous System Activity

Increased sympathetic nervous system activity is a well described feature of aging. By increasing peripheral resistance, this may be a contributory cause to the increased prevalence of hypertension in older people, although the progressive rise in systolic blood pressure also appears to be related to the development of increasing vascular stiffness [32]. Increases in total peripheral resistance with age are also mediated by a change in the balance of vasoconstrictor (maintained α-adrenergic and endothelin activity) as opposed to vasodilator (reduced nitric oxide release, reduced β_2-activity) influences. Aerobic exercise training and a low salt diet, in addition to enhancing β-adrenergic responsiveness also reduces resting sympathetic nervous system activity, which may be beneficial in management of hypertension and heart failure in older people [33].

Autonomic Dysfunction in Association with Central Nervous System Disease

Parkinson's disease and Alzheimer's disease have significant effects on autonomic nervous system physiology in older people, which further impair cardiovascular control. Reduced baroreflex sensitivity has been described in patients with Parkinson's or Alzheimer's disease [34] and abnormalities in parasympathetic function have been reported in patients with Alzheimer's disease [35]. Cardiac sympathetic denervation occurs in Parkinson's disease contributing to impaired autonomic control of blood pressure during postural changes [36]. The combined effects of aging and Parkinson's disease on baroreflex sensitivity result in a high prevalence of orthostatic hypotension when dopamine agonists are prescribed, frequently not recognized by patients or their doctors unless systematically examined for [37]. The high prevalence of hypotensive disorders likely contributes to the high prevalence of falls, and hip fracture, reported in these groups of patients.

Summary

Age-associated changes in autonomic physiology have profound effects on cardiovascular regulation, which may have secondary consequences in increasing risk of cerebrovascular disease. Changes in response to drug therapy, most notably β-adrenoceptor agonists and antagonists, need to be considered when prescribing to older people, but alterations in pharmacodynamic responsiveness to many drugs acting on the autonomic nervous system have not been well studied in detail for many drug groups. Degenerative dementias, and Parkinson's disease have further major effects on autonomic regulation and drug responsiveness, which need to be considered in prescribing cardiovascular drugs. Further research is needed to determine the effect of interventional strategies, such as exercise training and diet in maintaining autonomic function in old age, and the implications of altered autonomic function, in particular blood pressure regulation, to maintenance of health and risk of vascular disease and dementia in old age.

References

1   Prescriptions dispensed in the community. Statistics for 1989 to 1999: England. Statistical Bulletin. Department of Health. August 2000.
2   Ford GA, Blaschke TF, Hoffman BB: Pharmacodynamics; in George CG, Woodhouse K, MacLennan W, Denham M (eds): Drug Therapy in Old Age. London, Wiley & Sons, 1998, pp 59–72.
3   Vestal RE, Wood AJ, Shand DG: Reduced beta-adrenoceptor sensitivity in the elderly. Clin Pharmacol Ther 1979;26:181–186.
4   Ford GA, James OFW: Effects of autonomic blockade on cardiac β-adrenergic chronotropic responsiveness in healthy young, healthy elderly and endurance trained elderly subjects. Clin Sci 1994;87:297–302.

5   Poldermans D, Boersma E, Fioretti PM, van Urk H, Boomsma F, Man in't Veld AJ: Cardiac chronotropic responsiveness to beta-adrenoceptor stimulation is not reduced in the elderly. J Am Coll Cardiol 1995;25:995–999.

6   Lakatta EG, Sollott SJ: Perspectives on mammalian cardiovascular aging: Humans to molecules. Comp Biochem Physiol A Mol Integr Physiol 2002;132:699–721.

7   Feldman RD: A low-sodium diet corrects the defect in beta-adrenergic response in older subjects. Circulation 1992;85:612–618.

8   Iaccarino G, Cipolletta E, Fiorillo A, Annecchiarico M, Ciccarelli M, Cimini V, Koch WJ, Trimarco B: Beta(2)-adrenergic receptor gene delivery to the endothelium corrects impaired adrenergic vasorelaxation in hypertension. Circulation 2002;106:349–355.

9   Connolly MJ, Crowley JJ, Charan NB, Nielson CP, Vestal RE: Impaired bronchodilator response to albuterol in healthy elderly men and women. Chest 1995;108:401–406.

10   Lindholm LH, Ibsen H, Dahlof B, Devereux RB, Beevers G, de Faire U, Fyhrquist F, Julius S, Kjeldsen SE, Kristiansson K, Lederballe-Pedersen O, Nieminen MS, Omvik P, Oparil S, Wedel H, Aurup P, Edelman J, Snapinn S: The LIFE Study Group. Cardiovascular morbidity and mortality in patients with diabetes in the Losartan Intervention For Endpoint reduction in hypertension study (LIFE): A randomised trial against atenolol. Lancet 2002;359:1004–1010.

11   Messerli FH, Grossman E, Goldbourt U: Are beta-blockers efficacious as first-line therapy for hypertension in the elderly? A systematic review. JAMA 1998;279:1903–1907.

12   Brierley EJ, Broughton DL, James OFW, Alberti KG: Reduced awareness of hypoglycaemia in the elderly despite and intact counter-regulatory response. Q J Med 1995;88:439–445.

13   Gribbin B, Pickering TG, Sleight P: Decrease in baroreflex sensitivity with increasing arterial pressure and with increasing age. Br Heart J 1969;31:792.

14   Ford GA: Ageing and the baroreflex. Age Ageing 1999;28:337–338.

15   Monahan KD, Dinenno FA, Tanaka H, Clevenger CM, DeSouza CA, Seals DR: Regular aerobic exercise modulates age-associated declines in cardiovagal baroreflex sensitivity in healthy men. J Physiol 2000;529:263–271.

16   Bowman AJ, Clayton RH, Murray A, Reed JW, Subhan MF, Ford GA: Baroreflex function in sedentary and endurance trained elderly persons. Age Ageing 1997;26:289–294.

17   Robertson DR, Waller DG, Renwick AG, George CF: Age-related changes in the pharmaco-kinetics and pharmacodynamics of nifedipine. Br J Clin Pharmacol 1988;25:297–305.

18   Schoenberger JA: Drug-induced orthostatic hypotension. Drug Saf 1991;6:402–407.

19   Burrell LM, Johnston CI: Angiotensin II receptor antagonists. Potential in elderly patients with cardiovascular disease. Drugs Aging 1997;10:421–434.

20   Hata Y, Muratani H, Kimura Y, Fukiyama K, Kawano Y, Ashida T, Yokouchi M, Imai Y, Ozawa T, Fujii J, Omae T: Office blood pressure variability as a predictor of acute myocardial infarction in elderly patients receiving antihypertensive therapy. J Hum Hypertens 2002;16:141–146.

21   Kukla C, Sander D, Schwarze J, Wittich I, Klingelhofer J: Changes of circadian blood pressure patterns are associated with the occurrence of lacunar infarction. Arch Neurol 1998;55:683–688.

22   Eigenbrodt ML, Rose KM, Couper DJ, Arnett DK, Smith R, Jones D: Orthostatic hypotension as a risk factor for stroke: The Atheroscelrosis Risk In Communities (ARIC) study, 1987–1996. Stroke 2000;31:2307–2313.

23   Rose KM, Tyroler HA, Nardo CJ, et al: Orthostatic hypotension and the incidence of coronary heart disease: The Atherosclerosis Risk In Communitites study. Am J Hypertens 2000;13:571–578.

24   Ballard C, O'Brien J, Barber B, Scheltens P, Shaw F, McKeith I, Kenny RA: Neurocardiovascular instability, hypotensive episodes, and MRI lesions in neurodegenerative dementia. Ann N Y Acad Sci 2000;903:442–445.

25   Kario K, Eguchi K, Hoshide S, Hoshide Y, Umeda Y, Mitsuhashi T, Shimada K: U-curve relationship between orthostatic blood pressure change and silent cerebrovascular disease in elderly hypertensives: Orthostatic hypertension as a new cardiovascular risk factor. J Am Coll Cardiol 2002;40:133–141.

26   Mosqueda-Garcia R, Furlan R, Tank J, Fernandez-Violante R: The elusive pathophysiology of neurally mediated syncope. Circulation 2000;102:2898–2906.

27   Davies AJ, Steen N, Kenny RA: Carotid sinus hypersensitivity is common in older patients presenting to an accident and emergency department with unexplained falls. Age Ageing 2001;30:289–293.

28 Ward CR, McIntosh S, Kenny RA: Carotid sinus hypersensitivity – A modifiable risk factor for fractured neck of femur. Age Ageing 1999;28:127–133.

29 Mosqueda-Garcia R, Furlan R, Fernandez-Violante R, Desai T, Snell M, Jarai Z, Ananthram V, Robertson RM, Robertson D: Sympathetic and baroreceptor reflex function in neurally mediated syncope evoked by tilt. J Clin Invest 1997;99:2736–2744.

30 O'Mahony D: Pathophysiology of carotid sinus hypersensitivity in elderly patients. Lancet 1995;346:950–952.

31 Cole CR, Zuckerman J, Levine BD: Carotid sinus 'irritability' rather than hypersensitivity: A new name for an old syndrome? Clin Auton Res 2001;11:109–113.

32 Esler M, Rumantir M, Kaye D, Jennings G, Hastings J, Socratous F, Lambert G: Sympathetic nerve biology in essential hypertension. Clin Exp Pharmacol Physiol 2001;28:986–989.

33 Brown MD, Dengel DR, Hogikyan RV, Supiano MA: Sympathetic activity and the heterogeneous blood pressure response to exercise training in hypertensives. J Appl Physiol. 2002;92:1434–1442.

34 Szili-Torok T, Kalman J, Paprika D, Dibo G, Rozsa Z, Rudas L: Depressed baroreflex sensitivity in patients with Alzheimer's and Parkinson's disease. Neurobiol Aging 2001;22:435–438.

35 Wang SJ, Liao KK, Fuh JL, Lin KN, Wu ZA, Liu CY, Liu HC: Cardiovascular autonomic functions in Alzheimer's disease. Age Ageing 1994;23:400–404.

36 Goldstein DS, Holmes C, Li ST, Bruce S, Metman LV, Cannon RO 3rd: Cardiac sympathetic denervation in Parkinson disease. Ann Intern Med 2000;133:338–347.

37 Kujawa K, Leurgans S, Raman R, Blasucci L, Goetz CG: Acute orthostatic hypotension when starting dopamine agonists in Parkinson's disease. Arch Neurol 2000;57:1461–1463.

Gary A. Ford
Wolfson Unit of Clinical Pharmacology
Claremont Place, University of Newcastle upon Tyne, NE2 4HH (UK)
Tel. +44 191 222 7744, Fax +44 191 222 5827, E-Mail g.a.ford@ncl.ac.uk

Kuchel GA, Hof PR (eds): Autonomic Nervous System in Old Age.
Interdiscipl Top Gerontol. Basel, Karger, 2004, vol 33, pp 32–44

....

Normal and Pathological Changes in Cardiovascular Autonomic Function with Age

Preeti Attavar, David I. Silverman

Cardiology Division, University of Connecticut Health Center,
Farmington, Conn., USA

The effects of aging on the autonomic nervous system are multiple and vary between and within both sympathetic and parasympathetic portions. Normal human aging is associated with changes in autonomic control of several bodily functions, particularly those served by cardiovascular and thermoregulatory systems (table 1). Because the autonomic nervous system facilitates adaptation to physiologic stress, autonomic insufficiency in the elderly may not reveal itself under 'normal' resting conditions, yet may occur in response to changes in homeostasis. Common clinical manifestations of autonomic dysfunction in elderly patients, such as postural or postprandial hypotension, hypothermia and stroke, seldom occur in healthy individuals under the usual demands of daily life, but may become manifest during exposure to a variety of external influences, such as medications, changes in fluid intake, or environmental temperature changes.

Normal Changes in Cardiovascular Function

Heart Rate

Resting heart rate decreases with increasing age [1, 2]. Although heart rate is under combined sympathetic and parasympathetic control [3], parasympathetic influences predominate in human subjects under resting conditions. Electrophysiologic studies have demonstrated a progressive decline in both sinoatrial conduction and sinus node recovery time with aging. In the sinus node, the number of cells declines continuously; by 75 years of age, only 10%

Table 1. Age-related neurohumoral changes in the elderly

Increased sympathetic nerve activity
Impaired parasympathetic nerve activity
Decreased baroreflex sensitivity
Increase in plasma catecholamine (noradrenaline) levels
Impaired β-adrenergic receptor response to sympathetic stimulation

of the cells (approximately) that were present at 20 years of age remain [4]. The concomitant decline in heart rate variability with aging [5] is most likely due to reduced tone [6, 7]. Reliable noninvasive cardiovascular reflex tests of autonomic function, including heart rate responses to the Valsalva maneuver [8], deep breathing, and standing, all regress linearly with increasing age. Attenuated respiratory sinus arrhythmia with advancing age suggests a decrease in parasympathetic influence on sinus node function [9]. Blunted baroreceptor reflex response, which has been observed in animal models [10, 11] may contribute to sinus node depression, carotid sinus syndrome and syncope in the elderly.

Blood Pressure

Normal human aging is associated with several changes in autonomic regulation of blood pressure. Blood pressure is the product of heart rate, stroke volume, and systemic vascular resistance, all of which are regulated on a beat-to-beat basis by baroreflexes in both sympathetic and parasympathetic limbs of the autonomic nervous system. Age-related increases in both catecholamine plasma concentrations [12] and in the basal rate of sympathetic neural firing [13] reflect increased sympathetic nerve activity and suggest that blunted sinoaortic baroreflex sensitivity reduces the restraint on sympathetic outflow. Preservation of the sympathetic limb of the baroreflex with advancing age in turn suggests reduced tonic baroreceptor function (i.e. less inhibitory afferent signals at a given arterial pressure) but maintained gain during arterial pressure perturbations. In contrast, the heart rate reflex response to alterations in arterial pressure is clearly impaired with advancing age [14].

Normal human aging is associated with a reduction in baroreflex sensitivity (table 2). It has been suggested that the decrease in arterial distensibility that accompanies aging [15] and hypertension results in diminished baroreceptor center activity, and increased sympathetic outflow. Increased sympathetic outflow results in increased circulating noradrenaline, which in turn may result in further vasoconstriction, blood pressure elevation, and baroreflex impairment [16]. Age-related autonomic and baroreflex dysfunction may compromise arterial pressure homeostasis in response to diuretic therapy, altered fluid intake

Table 2. Physiologic and pathological mechanisms of hypotension in the elderly

Decreased baroreflex sensitivity
Impaired relaxation abnormality resulting in decreased early cardiac filling
Impaired regulation of intravascular volume status
Impaired β-adrenergic receptor response of inotropy and chronotropy
Impaired noradrenaline response to posture
Impaired α-adrenergic vascular response

and postural stress [17, 18]. Evidence suggests that basal plasma noradrenaline levels increase with age [19], while plasma adrenaline levels remain unaffected. The persistently blunted heart rate response that occurs in elderly subjects during hypotensive stress in the setting of prolonged and elevated plasma noradrenaline levels suggests that aging results in impaired β-adrenergic receptor responses to sympathetic activation [20, 21]. Maintenance of normal blood pressure also depends on the ability to generate an adequate cardiac output. Cardiac output at rest had been reported to decrease with normal aging [22, 23], while other studies using different selection or study criteria discovered little or no change in resting cardiac output or index with aging [23]. In contrast, the ability of older individuals to increase cardiac output and index in response to exercise is often diminished [24]. This decline is due not only to a reduction in heart rate response to β-adrenergic stimulation, but also to changes in systolic and diastolic cardiac performance that influence stroke volume [25].

Systolic Function
While myocardial contractile strength is preserved with advancing age, left-ventricular ejection fraction decreases in response to exertion [26]. This seemingly paradoxical response is due to a simultaneous reduction in β-adrenergic reactivity and an increase in afterload. Afterload increases progressively because of increased stiffening of the ascending aorta and narrowing of the peripheral vasculature. These changes result in increased systolic blood pressure and decreased maximum cardiac output during exercise. During exercise, one observes a striking decrease in heart rate and contractile response, as reflected by decreases in peak heart rate and peak ejection fraction, and by a progressively blunted exercise-induced decrease in end-systolic volume [27]. Stroke volume is preserved largely as the result of enhancement of the Frank-Starling mechanism; peak end-diastolic volume during exercise increases progressively with advancing age and is considerably larger in old than in young individuals. This augmentation of end-diastolic volume maintains stroke volume but attenuates the increase in ejection fraction.

Table 3. Hemodynamic response to exercise

Parameter	Young	Old
Heart rate	↑	↓
Ejection fraction	↑	↓
Cardiac output	↑	↓
Stroke volume	↑	↑
Left-ventricular size	↓	↑
Left-ventricular end-diastolic volume	↓	↑
Left-ventricular end-systolic volume	↓	↑
Systemic vascular resistance	↓	↑
Systolic blood pressure	↑	↑
Myocardial contractility	↑	↓

The age-associated decline in maximal heart rate and left-ventricular contractility during vigorous exercise probably reflects diminished β-adrenergic modulation of contractility, chronotropy and vasomotor tone (table 3). A similar mechanism can be demonstrated in young subjects in the presence of β-adrenergic blockade, suggesting that the age effect is due to reduced β-adrenergic responsiveness. This finding supports the hypothesis that blunted β-adrenergic receptor responsiveness underlies the attenuated increases in heart rate and myocardial contractility, and the cardiac dilation that occurs during exhaustive exercise in older individuals [25].

The clinical implications of blunted β-adrenergic receptor responsiveness with advancing age are considerable. The young respond to increased flow demands primarily with sympathoadrenergic activation, followed by β-adrenergic receptor-mediated modulation of cardiovascular performance. Such a mechanism maintains heart size despite increases in heart rate, venous return and systolic arterial pressure. As preload reserve is preserved, additional flow demands can be met by activation of the Frank-Starling mechanism, i.e. by increasing end-diastolic volume. In contrast, in the elderly, the increased peripheral flow demand is met primarily by activation of the preload reserve. As no further compensatory mechanism exists, additional flow demands may result in cardiovascular insufficiency. Such reduced cardiovascular reserve capacity may explain in part the higher incidence of acute and chronic heart failure in the elderly. The cardiovascular response to exercise in the elderly is comparable to disease states such as congestive heart failure, and emphasizes the importance of peripheral vasodilatation.

Diastolic Function

As a result of several structural and functional changes in the myocardium, the aging heart stiffens [28]. The resulting impairment in early diastolic ventricular filling results in prolongation of ventricular relaxation time, elevated end-diastolic volume, and higher cardiac filling pressures [29]. The age-related impairment in early ventricular filling makes the heart dependent on adequate preload to fill the ventricle, and in particular upon atrial contraction during late diastole to maintain stroke volume. Thus, orthostatic hypotension and syncope occur commonly in older people as a result of volume contraction or venous pooling (which reduce preload), or at the onset of atrial fibrillation when the atrial contribution to ventricular filling is suddenly lost.

An adequate blood pressure also depends on the maintenance of intra-vascular volume. Aging is associated with a progressive decline in plasma renin, angiotensin, and aldosterone levels [30]. These changes combined with elevations in atrial natriuretic peptide levels tend to promote salt wasting by the kidneys [30]. Any sodium depletion may impair the Frank-Starling mechanism on which the elderly depend to maintain cardiac output and arterial pressure during various forms of cardiovascular challenge. Thus, dehydration and hypotension may develop rapidly during conditions such as an acute illness, preparation of medical procedure, exposure to warm climate, when insensible fluid losses are increased and when patients are on diuretics. The interaction between volume contraction and impaired diastolic function may decrease cardiac output and result in hypotension, organ ischemia and syncope.

Diagnosis and Management for Specific Cardiovascular Diseases Related to Autonomic Dysfunction

Therapy for autonomic-related cardiac dysfunction in elderly patients should focus upon stabilization of symptoms, improvement in quality of life, practicality of administration, and established efficacy. The geriatric physician constantly wrestles with the paradox that most medical therapies are tested in middle-aged or 'young old' patients, and that treatment efficacy is then extrapolated to populations whose baseline characteristics differ markedly from enrolled subjects. Response to therapy, in terms of pharmacokinetics, efficacy, and adverse effects, however, is heterogeneous, and direct transfer of treatment principles derived from nonequivalent groups of patients confers its own set of hazards. Furthermore, improved survival, the classic outcome variable by which therapeutics are commonly judged, may have less applicability in older patients approaching a maximum lifespan.

Autonomic dysfunction in elderly patients is usually multifactorial in etiology, and may be the product of the intersection of both natural aging and disease states that alter normal autonomic nervous system function, such as diabetes induced peripheral neuropathy, intrinsic conduction system disease, and heart failure. Loss of any part of the normal reflexes that control basic cardiovascular functions such as reaction to change in posture and response to exercise produce a variety of symptoms that may defy ready categorization and straightforward management.

Syncope

The most obvious clinical problem in this arena is syncope. While cardiogenic syncope remains the most common and most life-threatening form of this disorder, noncardiogenic syncope produces substantial disability for patients and ongoing frustration for clinicians. Once again, determining the difference between a normal aging response and true pathology remains a formidable challenge in the work-up of this problem. Traditionally, investigation of syncope has focused upon identification of a dysrhythmic cause, including malignant ventricular tachycardia supraventricular tachycardia, or symptomatic bradycardia (fig. 1).

A thorough history in the determination of an etiology of syncope is critically important if a timely and accurate diagnosis is to be made. The difficulty of determining whether or not true syncope has occurred represents a formidable challenge for any clinician. Often the circumstances surrounding the episode (time of day, posture, level of activity) will provide as much information as any account of the event itself. Time course from onset of symptoms to actual loss of consciousness is perhaps the most critical historical detail, since most forms of neurocardiogenic syncope are preceded by at least some degree of premonition or have a positional component, while arrhythmogenic syncope classically presents as a sudden, unanticipated event. Precipitating factors, such as change in position, sudden emotion, or pain all suggest an autonomic component, while physical exertion preceding syncope can herald either ischemic-induced arrhythmia or left-ventricular outflow obstruction if symptoms ensue shortly after cessation of exercise. The value of a witnessed account cannot be overemphasized, since patients suffering from syncope may provide little or no account of the event, and will often be unable to provide any information regarding the length of the episode. The experience of witnesses must be considered in evaluating their account, as trained professionals, such as nurses, law enforcement officers, or paramedics, can generally be expected to provide more accurate information. Distinguishing between transient seizure activity related to hypoxia and true seizures requires attention to accompanying signs such as tongue biting, postictal state, incontinence, and lactic acidosis.

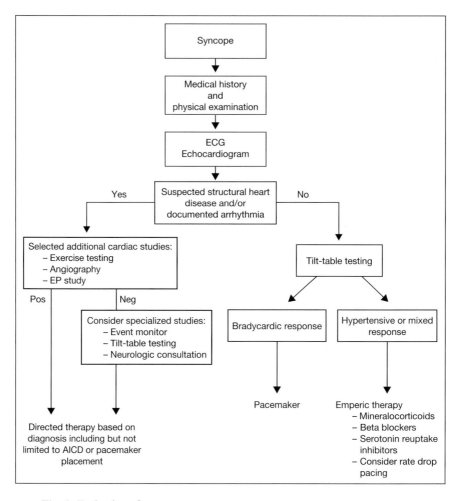

Fig. 1. Evaluation of syncope.

Physical exam plays a crucial role in developing a differential diagnosis, as it provides a rationale for further testing, and guides choices for therapy [31]. Fundamental elements of the cardiovascular exam that deserve emphasis include vital signs (especially orthostatic heart rate and blood pressure) palpation of the carotid pulse (parvus et tardus in aortic stenosis), direct observation of the neck veins (elevated in cor pulmonale or heart failure), cardiac auscultation (for the systolic ejection murmur of aortic stenosis or hypertrophic obstructive cardio-myopathy), examination of the extremities (for evidence of peripheral neuro-pathy or vascular insufficiency), and selected neurological exam including evidence of gait, strength, or abnormalities of balance.

Further testing should proceed with an evaluation of cardiac function, preferably by transthoracic (surface) echocardiography. The preponderance of data suggest that underlying left-ventricular function plays such an important role in determination of prognosis in the setting of syncope that it provides the first logical step in any evaluation of the syncopal or presyncopal patient. Mechanical causes of syncope, including aortic stenosis, hypertrophic obstructive cardiomyopathy, and severe pulmonary hypertension, are readily established or excluded by echocardiography [32]. The presence of focal wall motion abnormalities establishes the diagnosis of ischemic heart disease in the absence of any previous documentation of myocardial infarction or angina, and readily categorizes the syncopal patient as high risk for malignant ventricular arrhythmia [33]. The likelihood of recurrent syncopal episodes in such patients is markedly increased compared to those with normal left-ventricular function or minor abnormalities.

Although 24-hour Holter monitoring remains a frequently ordered test in patients with syncope, the limitations of Holter monitoring have become increasingly appreciated as the heterogeneous nature of syncope became clearer. The best available data suggest that Holter monitoring provides limited sensitivity for identification of either malignant ventricular arrhythmia or bradycardia, in part because of the frequency of unrelated rhythm disturbances in the elderly [34]. For patients with a high index of suspicion for malignant arrhythmia, programmed electrical stimulation has largely replaced holter monitoring as the diagnostic procedure of choice for identification and characterization of the abnormal rhythm. The combination of coronary artery disease, inducible ventricular tachycardia, and decreased left-ventricular systolic function produces a subset of patients at high risk for recurrent events and sudden cardiac death [35]. Events and mortality in such patients defined by these characteristics are significantly reduced by the placement of an automatic implantable cardioverter-defibrillator, and such device placement has become the standard of care for cardiac syncope when inducibility and/or high risk substrate is established [36].

Bradycardic causes of syncope include high degree carotid sinus hypersensitivity, atrioventricular block, asystole, or sick sinus syndrome. When bradycardic syncope is suspected in the absence of documentation, event monitoring using a portable device may provide a diagnosis. Provocative carotid sinus massage can yield the diagnosis of carotid hypersensitivity in selected cased. In some patients, invasive recording of sinus node function including sinus node recovery time may also yield a diagnosis. For patients with symptomatic, documented bradycardia, pacemaker therapy is curative, and further management revolves around choice of pacing mode (dual vs. single chamber, with or without activity response, with or without mode switching). While indications for pacemaker placement are long established, the ever-increasing array of pacing technologies presents an often-bewildering surfeit of choices once the decision for pacemaker placement has been made. Reasonable attention may be paid to the incremental value of added technology and the cost/benefit ratio thereof. Patients with combined tachycardia-bradycardia may require a combination of atrioventricular nodal blocking agents including β-blockers, α calcium channel blockers, as well as digoxin for control of their supraventricular arrhythmia and pacing for suppression of the resultant hypersensitivity to these agents.

For patients in whom the presence of malignant arrhythmia or a mechanical cause has been excluded, the value of tilt table testing in older patients is the subject of ongoing controversy. Neurocardiogenic syncope had been previously thought to be a diagnosis largely restricted to younger patients, but more recent data suggest that tilt testing produces a surprisingly high yield in appropriately selected patients. In a series of 176 patients age >65 (with 43 patients age >80), 34% of patients had a positive tilt table test using a standard protocol (45 min of upright tilt followed by 15 min of isoproterenol infusion), compared to 45% of patients <65 years old [37].

Despite advances in diagnosis, treatment of neurocardiogenic syncope depends upon an empiric approach based upon interruption of the one or more portions of the enhanced autonomic response that promotes the syndrome. Various modalities may produce symptom improvement, including β-adrenergic receptor antagonists and mineralocorticoids. Therapy should be administered stepwise, with careful monitoring for symptom improvement and adverse effects. Patients with documented carotid hypersensitivity should avoid potential stimuli such as tight collars.

Heart Failure and Altered Neurohumoral Response
The last 20 years have produced a revolution in our understanding of heart failure and in its management. Previously believed to be a hemodynamic issue primarily related to inadequate cardiac output, heart failure is now recognized as a 'misguided' neurohumoral response to the stimuli that inadequate cardiac output produces. The normally adaptive response to hemorrhage includes α-adrenergic induced peripheral vasoconstriction, β-adrenergic induced contractility with increased chronotropy, angiotensin-induced renal vasoconstriction, plus aldosterone and antidiuretic hormone-induced salt and water retention. These responses preserve circulatory volume and are life-saving when the patient is bleeding, but in the setting of heart failure provide short-term improvement while accelerating long-term deterioration and hastening death. The descending spiral of vasoconstriction, increased salt and water retention, consequent edema and pulmonary congestion results in a worsening of symptoms [38]. Increased catecholamine levels, well documented in heart failure [39]

improve short-term function at the expense of excessive energy expenditure, enhanced cell destruction [40], and potentially fatal proarrhythmia [41].

Many elderly patients suffer from multiple conditions that produce symptoms similar to those caused by heart failure, or exacerbate heart failure symptoms that are already present. In particular, a careful effort should be made to identify concomitant pulmonary disease, especially if the diagnosis of heart failure remains uncertain. While the clinical diagnosis of heart failure is established via history, physical exam, and chest X-ray, baseline assessment of ejection fraction represents a critical next step prior to or simultaneous with clinical management. Radionucleotide ventriculography (RVG) and echocardiography represent competing technologies that offer assessment of ventricular architecture and function; the chief advantage of RVG is its routine quantitation of ejection, echocardiography by comparison offers a detailed assessment that often leads to identification of the underlying abnormality. Regional wall motion abnormalities consistent with ischemic heart disease, valvular abnormalities consistent with stenosis and/or regurgitation, and hypertrophy, consistent with abnormal relaxation, are all readily identifiable by routine echocardiographs.

Diastolic dysfunction continues to be an underappreciated cause of heart failure. The presence of documented pulmonary congestion in the absence of systolic dysfunction has been proposed as a new clinical definition of diastolic heart failure [42], but even this classification would not exclude less common causes of abnormal relaxation such as restrictive cardiomyopathy. Multiple echocardiographic signs of diastolic dysfunction have been reported, but echocardiography remains a problematic tool for making the diagnosis, since many echocardiographic findings that suggest diastolic dysfunction in younger patients, such as abnormal mitral inflow patterns, are universally altered in the elderly.

Therapy should begin with appropriate lifestyle intervention including dietary modification of salt intake, careful daily monitoring of weight for accelerating fluid elimination, and modest regular exercise whenever possible. Underlying causes for myopathy such as hemochromatosis and thyroid disease should be considered if the cause of heart failure is not otherwise obvious. Correction of any underlying structural abnormalities that will substantially improve or resolve the underlying heart failure should be carefully considered for some patients. Aortic valve replacement, for instance is definitive therapy for patients with symptomatic critical aortic stenosis. Patients with evidence for viable but nonfunctional regions of the left ventricle ('hibernating' myocardium) should be carefully evaluated as revascularization can, in some patients, lead to dramatic improvement. Ischemic heart disease should be treated with appropriate lifestyle modification and, where appropriate, risk factor intervention including lipid, glucose, and blood pressure control. Smoking cessation should be encouraged in the strongest possible terms, and all available therapies for smoking cessation should be explored.

Drug therapy centers on interruption of the neurohumoral response. Initial therapy in the setting of decompensated heart failure begins with relief of pulmonary congestion and edema via loop diuretics administered intravenously, along with oxygen and short-acting nitrates when appropriate. Angiotensin-converting enzyme inhibitors represent the bedrock of therapy, and should be initiated as soon as the diagnosis is confirmed. Despite their efficacy, β-blockers require stabilization of heart failure before they may be initiated, and careful dose titration is required. Spironolactone represents an important new advance in heart failure therapy, and should be considered standard adjunctive therapy. Despite its null effect upon survival, digoxin provides measurable symptom relief for selected patients with advanced symptoms. Long-term anticoagulation may reduce thromboembolic risk in patients whose Heart failure occurs in the setting of left-ventricular dilatation.

The paradox that most appropriately treated heart failure patients die arrhythmic deaths, while most antiarrhythmics dramatically shorten survival, remains a sobering lesson. Because of their complex and hazardous effects, only an expert should prescribe antiarrhythmic drugs. In general, benign ventricular ectopy, including ventricular premature systoles, bigeminy, or even couplets, has limited prognostic significance and should not be suppressed. When ectopy is complex, amiodarone can be given with reasonable safety, but routine safety monitoring for pulmonary, thyroid and hepatic toxicity is required. In patients with ischemic heart disease with malignant, symptomatic ventricular ectopy, or with reproducible ventricular tachycardia in the setting of systolic dysfunction, implantable carioverter-defibrillators have been shown to prevent sudden death and improve survival.

In conclusion, normal autonomic function plays a critical role in the maintenance of cardiovascular health. At the same time, autonomic dysfunction contributes substantially to the development and progression of cardiovascular disease in old age. Remembering that autonomic dysfunction most commonly reveals itself during periods of stress may be crucial in making the distinction between 'normal' decline in cardiovascular autonomic function and pathologic deterioration. Treatment 'norms' established in younger populations must often be modified when selecting the threshold for intervention. Finally, attention to quality as much as duration of life should remain a fundamental goal of therapy.

References

1   Howell TH: The pulse rate in old age. J Gerontol 1948;3:272–275.
2   Gautschy B, Weidmann P, Gnadinger MP: Autonomic function tests as related to age and gender in normal man. Klin Wochenschr 1986;64:499–505.

3   Vita G, Princi P, Calabro R, Toscano A, Manna L, Messina C: Cardiovascular reflex tests. Assessment of age-adjusted normal range. J Neurol Sci 1986;75:263–274.

4   Davies MJ: Pathology of the conduction system; in Caird FL, Dalle JLC, Kennedy RD (eds): Cardiology in Old Age. New York, Plenum Press, 1976, pp 57–59.

5   Waddington JL, MacCulloch MJ, Sambrooks JL: Resting heart rate variability declines with age. Experientia 1979;35:1197–1198.

6   Dauchot P, Gravenstein JS: Effects of atropine on the electrocardiogram in different age groups. Clin Pharmacol Ther 1971;12:274–280.

7   Nalefski LA, Brown CFG: Action of atropine on the cardiovascular system in normal persons. Arch Intern Med 1950;86:898–907.

8   Shimada K, Kitazumi T, Ogura H, Sadakane N, Ozawa T: Effects of age and blood pressure on the cardiovascular responses to the Valsalva maneuver. J Am Geriatr Soc 1986;34: 431–434.

9   Seals DR, Taylor JA, Ng AV, Esler MD: Exercise and aging: Autonomic control of the circulation. Med Sci Sports Exercise 1994;26:568–576.

10   Hajduczok G, Chapleau MW, Abboud FM: Increase in sympathetic activity with age. II. Role of impairment of cardiopulmonary baroreflexes. Am J Physiol 1991;260:H1121–H1127.

11   Hajduczok G, Chapleau MW, Johnson SL, Abboud FM: Increase in sympathetic activity with age. I. Role of impairment of arterial baroreflexes. Am J Physiol 1991;260:H1113–H1120.

12   Esler MD, Turner AG, Kaye DM, et al: Aging effects on human sympathetic neuronal function. Am J Physiol 1995;268:R278–R285.

13   Ebert TJ, Morgan BJ, Barney JA, Denahan T, Smith JJ: Effects of aging on baroreflex regulation of sympathetic activity in humans. Am J Physiol 1992;263:H798–H803.

14   Gribbin B, Pickering TG, Sleight P, Peto R: Effect of age and high blood pressure on baroreflex sensitivity in man. Circ Res 1971;29:424–431.

15   Gozna ER, Marble AE, Shaw A, Holland JG: Age-related changes in the mechanics of the aorta and pulmonary artery of man. J Appl Physiol 1974;36:407–411.

16   Shimada K, Kitazumi T, Sadakane N, Ogura H, Ozawa T: Age-related changes of baroreflex function, plasma norepinephrine, and blood pressure. Hypertension 1985;7:113–117.

17   Shannon RP, Wei JY, Rosa RM, Epstein FH, Rowe JW: The effect of age and sodium depletion on cardiovascular response to orthostasis. Hypertension 1986;8:438–443.

18   Weinberger M, Fineberg NS: Sodium and volume sensitivity of blood pressure. Age and pressure change over time. Hypertension 1991;18:67–71.

19   Veith RC, Featherstone JA, Linares OA, Halter JB: Age differences in plasma norepinephrine kinetics in humans. J Gerontol 1986;41:319–324.

20   Stratton JR, Cerqueira MD, Schwartz RS, Levy WC, Veith RC, Kahn SE, Abrass IB: Differences in cardiovascular responses to isoproterenol in relation to age and exercise training in healthy men. Circulation 1992;86:504–512.

21   Vestal RE, Wood AJ, Shand DG: Reduced beta-adrenoceptor sensitivity in the elderly. Clin Pharmacol Ther 1979;26:181–186.

22   Brandfonbrener M, Landowne M, Shock NW: Changes in cardiac output with age. Circulation 1955;12:557–566.

23   Lakatta EG: Cardiovascular system; in Masoro EJ (ed): Aging. Oxford, Oxford University Press, 1995, vol 11, chap 17, p 413.

24   Mann DL, Denenberg BS, Gash AK, Makler PT, Bove AA: Effects of age on ventricular performance during graded supine exercise. Am Heart J 1986;111:108–115.

25   Rodeheffer RJ, Gerstenblith G, Becker LC, Fleg JL, Weisfeldt ML, Lakatta EG: Exercise cardiac output is maintained with advancing age in healthy human subjects: Cardiac dilatation and increased stroke volume compensate for a diminished heart rate. Circulation 1984;69: 203–213.

26   Julius S, Amery A, Whitlock LS, Conway J: Influence of age on the hemodynamic response to exercise. Circulation 1967;36:222–230.

27   Fleg JL, O'Connor FC, Gerstenblith G, Becker LC, Clulow J, Schulman SP, Lakatta EG: Impact of age on the cardiovascular response to dynamic upright exercise in healthy men and women. J Appl Physiol 1995;78:890–900.

28 Bonow RO, Vitale DF, Bacharach SL, Maron BJ, Green MV: Effects of aging on asynchronous left ventricular regional function and global ventricular filling in normal human subjects. J Am Coll Cardiol 1988;11:50–58.

29 Kitzman DW, Sheikh KH, Beere PA, Philips JL, Higginbotham MB: Age-related alterations of Doppler left ventricular filling indexes in normal subjects are independent of left ventricular mass, heart rate, contractility and loading conditions. J Am Coll Cardiol 1991;18:1243–1250.

30 Shannon RP, Minaker KL, Rowe JW: The influence of age on water balance in man. Semin Nephrol 1984;8:438–443.

31 Abrams J: Essentials of Cardiac Physical Diagnosis. Philadelphia, Lea & Febiger, 1987.

32 Benditt DG: Syncope; in Willerson JT, Cohn JN (eds): Cardiovascular Medicine. New York, Churchill Livingstone, 1995, pp 1404–1421.

33 Kapoor WN, Karpf M, Wierand S, Peterson JR, Levey GS: A prospective evaluation and follow-up of patients with syncope. N Engl J Med 1983;309:197–204

34 Fleg JL, Kennedy HL: Cardiac arrhythmias in a healthy elderly population: Detection by 24-hour ambulatory electrocardiography. Chest 1982;81:302–307.

35 DiMarco JP, Garan H, Harthorne JW, Ruskin JN: Intracardiac electrophysiologic techniques in recurrent syncope of unknown cause. Ann Intern Med 1981;95:542–548.

36 A comparison of antiarrhythmic-drug therapy with implantable defibrillators in patients resuscitated from near-fatal ventricular arrhythmias. The Antiarrhythmics versus Implantable Defibrillators (AVID) Investigators. N Engl J Med 1997;337:1576–1583.

37 Bloomfield D, Maurer M, Bigger JT Jr: Effects of age on outcome of tilt-table testing. Circulation 1967;36:222–230.

38 Katz AM: Physiology of the Heart, ed 2. New York, Raven Press, 1992, pp 638–668.

39 Cohn JN, Levine TB, Olivari MT, Garberg V, Lura D, Francis GS, Simon AB, Rector T: Plasma norepinephrine as a guide to prognosis in patients with chronic congestive heart failure. N Engl J Med 1984;311:819–823.

40 Katz AM, Silverman DI: Treatment of heart failure in the elderly. Hosp Pract 2000;35:19–31.

41 Bigger JT Jr: Why patients with congestive heart failure die: Arrhythmias and sudden cardiac death. Circulation 1987;75:IV28–IV35.

42 Vasan RS, Levy D: Defining diastolic heart failure: A call for standardized diagnostic criteria. Circulation 2000;101:2118–2121.

Preeti Attavar
Cardiology Division, University of Connecticut Health Center
263 Farmington Ave., Farmington, CT 06030–1305 (USA)
Tel. +1 860 679 2771, Fax +1 860 679 3346, E-Mail silverman@nso1.uchc.edu

Kuchel GA, Hof PR (eds): Autonomic Nervous System in Old Age.
Interdiscipl Top Gerontol. Basel, Karger, 2004, vol 33, pp 45–52

....

The Autonomic Nervous System and Blood Pressure Regulation in the Elderly

Edmund Bourke[a], James R. Sowers[b]

[a] Division of Endocrinology, Diabetes and Hypertension and Geriatrics Program at
   SUNY Health Science Center at Brooklyn, and VAMC, Brooklyn, N.Y., USA;
[b] University of Missouri-Columbia, Department of Internal Medicine, MA410,
   Health Sciences Center, Columbia, Mo., USA

Autonomic nervous system (ANS) function may be altered by advancing age, as well as by age-associated disease. Such changes may all contribute to impaired hemodynamic homeostasis in late life and may also influence the presentation and the management of specific diseases common in late life. For example, in contrast to younger subjects, hypertension in the elderly is often characterized hemodynamically by a low plasma volume and cardiac output in the setting of elevated total peripheral resistance. Additionally, the elderly have relatively increased adiposity and lesser skeletal muscle mass. The resultant insulin resistance/hyperinsulinemia then indirectly increases ANS function. The elderly are also more prone to orthostatic hypotension. Multiple factors contribute to an increased risk of orthostatic hypotension in the older individual including reductions in baroreceptor sensitivity, cardiac output and intravascular volume. Finally, aging is associated with alterations in the circadian control of a number of functions including sleep and ANS function. Thus, it is important to review both normal age-associated changes in the ANS, as well as changes in ANS function resulting from diseases that are more prevalent among the elderly.

Autonomic Nervous System Physiology

Norepinephrine (NE), epinephrine and dopamine are released by postganglionic sympathetic nerve terminals and the adrenal medulla. They then interact with cell surface receptor molecules in many diverse target organs including the cardiovascular tissues [1–7]. All three catecholamines are synthesized by a series of enzymatic steps, beginning with conversion of the amino acid tyrosine to dehydroxyphenylalanine (*L*-dopa) by the enzyme tyrosine hydroxylase through what is generally the rate-limiting step in catecholamine biosynthesis. The second and third steps in catecholamine biosynthesis are catalyzed by dopa-decarboxylase and dopamine β-hydroxylase (DβH), respectively. Phenylethanol-amine N-methyltransferase, the final enzyme involved in catecholamine biosynthesis converts NE to epinephrine. Activities of these enzymes are subject to both short- and long-term regulation by neural and by hormonal mechanisms. Catecholamines are released by exocytosis during stimulation of sympathetic nerves and chromaffin cells. A number of substances are released simultaneously with catecholamines during exocytosis. These include chromogranins, a family of proteins which localize to secretory granules in neuroendocrine cells, adenosine triphosphate (ATP) and DβH. Both circulating DβH and chromogranin, as well as NE, have been used as indirect indices of ANS activity. Neurotransmitter actions of catecholamines are terminated principally by neuronal reuptake.

Neuronally released NE undergoes one of three fates within the neuronal synapse: neuronal reuptake accounting for 80% of the released NE; uptake and metabolism by postsynaptic tissues with the consequent release of O-methylated metabolites in plasma and urine; or diffusion (spillover) from the synaptic cleft into the extracellular fluid. As potential differences exist among these three processes in persons with differing pathophysiologic states, NE spillover has been suggested as a more accurate index of ANS activity than measurement of plasma NE. Direct sympathetic neuronal recording (micro-neurographic measurements) is an even more precise measurement of ANS activity and has been increasingly used. Nevertheless, it appears that measurement of plasma NE levels is a relatively accurate index of ASN activity.

NE and epinephrine interact with cell surface adrenergic receptors divided into two classes: α- and β-receptors. These receptors mediate their effects via interaction with guanosine nucleotide-binding regulatory proteins (G proteins). These G proteins are coupled directly to ion channels or linked to a second messenger system (i.e., phosphoinositide hydrolysis and/or protein phosphorylation). Identification of their molecular structure and gene control has led to the identification of receptors in three families (α_{1ABC}, α_{2ABC} and $\beta_{1,2,3}$). α_1-adrenergic receptors are autoreceptors localized on postganglionic nerve terminals that synthesize NE. When activated by catecholamines, α_2-receptors inhibit further NE release. Activation of brain α_2-receptors reduces systemic sympathetic output. Activation of β_1-adrenergic receptors stimulates the rate and strength of cardiac contraction, lipolysis in fat cells, and renal renin production. The β_2-adrenergic receptor relaxes smooth muscle cells in the vasculature. The β_2-adrenergic receptor is downregulated with aging, by several possible mechanisms. One process that decreases β-adrenergic signaling involves phosphorylation of agonist-occupied receptors,

Table 1. Alterations in the cardiovascular hemodynamics of the elderly

1. Enhanced sympathetic nervous system activity
2. Decreased baroreceptor sensitivity
3. Increased peripheral vascular resistance
4. Tendency to lowered cardiac output
5. Tendency to contracted intravascular volume
6. Suppressed plasma renin activity
7. Decreased vascular endothelium production of nitric oxide
8. Increased blood pressure variability
9. Tendency to reduced renal blood flow

uncoupling of the receptors from G proteins, and internalization of receptors from the membrane into the cytoplasm. Regardless of the mechanism, downregulation of the β_2-adrenergic receptor with aging results in decreased β_2-adrenergic effects on the heart (reduced chrono- and inotrophic effects) on the juxtaglomerular cells (reduced renin production) and the vasculature (relatively unopposed α-adrenergic activity and increased vascular resistance) [8–10] (table 1).

Both sinoaortic high pressure and cardiopulmonary low pressure baroreceptors play an integral role in the regulation of ANS activity via regulation of the rostral ventrolateral reticular nucleus (RVL) sympathetic discharge [11–15]. The RVL neurons are the major source of tonic excitation of spinal preganglionic sympathetic neurons. Electrophysiologically, these neurons are spontaneously active and discharge with a rhythm tracking with the heart rate. The cardiac rhythmicity is imposed by their phasic inhibition by baroreceptor stimulation. Conversely, baroreceptor withdrawal activates these neurons. Baroreflexes are initiated in response to stimulation of pressure/stretch sensitive carotid and aortic and stretch sensitive cardiopulmonary baroreceptors. Baroreflex stimulation causes inhibition of sympathetic nerve activity, resulting in vasodilation, a fall of blood pressure, and a slowing of heart rate, the latter of which results from cardiovagal excitation and cardiosympathetic inhibition. Similarly, reduction or interruption of baroreceptor input elevates blood pressure by 'disinhibiting' RVL neurons and, in turn, increasing their excitation. Decreased baroreceptor sensitivity, as exists in hypertension and aging, leads to an increased variability of blood pressure as well as an altered circadian rhythm of blood pressure [10–14], as is often seen in the elderly (table 1).

Aging and the Autonomic Nervous System

In evaluating the status of the ANS in aging, one must consider the presence of multiple confounders that impact on ANS activity. With aging there is a propensity to a relatively increased fat to muscle ratio [16–18]. Increased relative obesity and hypertension are strongly positively associated at all ages. Increased insulin resistance and the consequent hyperinsulinemia may directly elevate sympathetic nervous system activity in the aging individual [16–18]. Thus, increased relative adiposity, hyperinsulinemia, hyperleptinemia and consequent hyperadrenergic state appear to be a critical link to age-related increase in blood pressure (table 1).

A number of investigations have shown that there is an age-associated increase in plasma NE levels [19–21] (table 1). Data from studies of tracer NE kinetics indicate that the primary determinant of the increase in plasma NE is an increase in the rate of NE spillover into the circulation, coupled with a decrease in the rate of NE clearance from the circulation [22, 23]. Results from studies of muscle sympathetic nerve activity of the peritoneal nerve have demonstrated an increase in muscle sympathetic nerve activity with aging [24]. When tracer NE kinetic studies have been performed to assess regional, organ specific ANS activity in older persons an age-associated increase in the rate of cardiac, but not renal, NE spillover has been observed.

Increased peripheral vascular resistance, the hallmark of hypertension associated with aging, reflects increased catecholamine exposure and altered tissue sensitivity. Indeed, relatively increased α-adrenoreceptor-mediated contraction versus β-mediated dilatation occurs with aging. Studies have demonstrated an age-related decline in isoproterenol-mediated dilatation of the brachial artery and hand veins. Cardiac responses to β-adrenergic receptor stimulation are impaired to the chronotrophic and contractility response to β-agonists. Indeed, there appears to be functional uncoupling of the β-adrenergic receptor from the catalytic unit of adenyl cyclase, with a decrease in the proportion of β-receptors in the high-affinity agonist-binding state [25]. The importance of the ANS in the pathophysiology of hypertension in the elderly is indicated by the strong association between plasma NE and systemic vascular resistance in aging persons. In the Normative Aging Studies, there was also a strong age-independent relationship between urinary NE excretion and blood pressure [26]. Finally, plasma epinephrine has also been reported to remain elevated in hypertensives beyond age 60 years, suggesting an age-related role of this catecholamine in sustaining inappropriately high ANS activity [27].

Increased relative adiposity and insulin resistance/hyperinsulinemia appear to be a driving force for enhanced ANS with advancing age [16–19]. Regulation of body fat stores is achieved through several mechanisms that form a negative feedback 'lipostat'; changes in adipose tissue mass are signaled to central nervous system (CNS) centers that regulate both appetite and energy expenditure. Leptin is a major factor produced by adipose tissue that acts in the CNS to regulate appetite and increase energy expenditure, in part, by increasing sympathetic nervous system activity [28, 29]. Aging in westernized, industrialized societies is often associated with a loss of lean body mass and an increase in adipose tissue, especially visceral fat [30–32]. This age-related increase in total body fat and central adiposity is greater in women than men [32]. Reductions in weight and body fat are associated with parallel reductions in ANS activity [16]. Further, regularly performed endurance exercise partially protects, but does not abolish, the increase in relative body fat with advancing age [33–35]. Further, exercise intervention studies [33, 35] have demonstrated that endurance training reduces central body fat, a parameter that is linked to insulin resistance and hyperinsulinemia. Thus, aerobic exercise may partly abolish the age-related increase in ANS activity through reductions in insulin and leptin as well as other mechanisms [36].

The elderly are more likely to experience orthostatic hypotension than their younger counterparts [36, 37]. The reasons for this propensity are multiple. For example, there is relative downregulation of β-adrenoreceptors, decreased cardiac output and decreased intravascular plasma volume [8–10]. There is also a diminution in baroreflex sensitivity, particularly that of the low-pressure cardio-pulmonary stretch receptors, which are very important in minute-to-minute regulation cardiovascular modulatory responses to change in posture [11–14]. Their reduction in sensitivity appears to be related to alteration in the afferent and central components of this reflex arc [13, 14]. This reduction in baroreflex sensitivity is especially relevant with respect to diminished ability of the elderly to maintain blood pressure homeostasis in response to volume depletion (i.e., with dehydration, bleeding or diuretic therapy) and in the face of vasodila-tory blood pressure medications (i.e., α-blockers and dihydropyridine calcium channel blockers) [36–39].

With advancing age, there is a propensity to greater fluctuations in blood pressures, especially systolic blood pressure. This is likely due, in part, to reductions in baroreflex sensitivity [40, 41]. There is also a propensity for a reduction of the degree of blood pressure reduction (dipping) at night time [40, 41]. This reduction in nocturnal blood pressure dipping is probably related to reduced baroreceptor sensitivity, alterations in sleep and altered renal afferent sympathetic input to the CNS [40, 41]. This is especially relevant for cardiovascular disease risk and stroke which have their highest frequency in the early hours of the morning prior to awakening. The practical caveats of these observations regarding greater variability of blood pressure, and loss of normal 'dipping' of blood pressure are inherently apparent. First, more blood pressure measurements are necessary to evaluate the most representative pressure, and the office blood pressures often underestimate the 24-hour pressure load to which cardiovascular, renal and cerebral vasculature systems are exposed.

The above observations regarding age-related alterations in ANS function have a number of practical ramifications in caring for the elderly. First, one should be aware that cardiac output and intravascular volume are reduced, thus making the elderly much more susceptible to orthostatic hypotension. Accordingly, therapies that further reduce cardiac output or intravascular volume should be administered very carefully in older subjects [37–39]. Blood pressures should be checked in the upright as well as supine position. Falls due to orthostatic hypotension lead to tremendous disability in the elderly [39]. Because of the greater variability of blood pressure, especially systolic blood pressure, more measurements are needed to ascertain the most representative blood pressures. Finally, because of enhanced ANS activity and reduced β-adrenoreceptor responses, enhanced peripheral vascular resistance is the hallmark of hypertension in the elderly [36–41].

Acknowledgement

The authors wish to thank Paddy McGowan for her excellent work in preparing this review. Dr. Sowers' research is supported by grants from the NIH HL66119–02, VA Merit Award 0018, and ADA RA0095.

References

1   Cooper JR, Bloom FE, Roth RE: The Biochemical Basis of Neuropharmacology. New York, Oxford University Press, 1991, pp 220–284.
2   Lefkowitz RJ, Hoffman BB, Taylor P: Neurohumoral transmission: The autonomic and somatic motor systems; in Goodman LS, Gibson A, Rall TW, Nies AS, Taylor P (eds): The Pharmacological Basis of Therapeutics, ed 8. New York, Pergamon Press, 1990, pp 84–121.
3   Esler M, Jennings G, Lambert G, Meredith I, Horne M, Eisenhofer G: Overflow of catecholamine neurotransmitters to the circulation: Source, fate; and functions. Physiol Rev 1990;70:763–785.
4   Insel PA: Seminars in medicine of the Beth Israel Hospital, Boston. Adrenergic receptors – Evolving concepts and clinical implications. N Engl J Med 1996;334:580–585.
5   Linares OA, Jacquez JA, Zech LA, Smith MJ, Sanfield JA, Morrow LA, Rosen SG, Halter JB: Norepinephrine metabolism in humans. J Clin Invest 1987;80:1332–1334.
6   Wallin BG, Morlin C, Hjemduhl P: Muscle sympathetic activity and venous plasma noradrenaline concentrations during static exercise in normotensive and hypertensive subjects. Acta Physiol Scand 1987;129:489–497.
7   Eisenhofer G, Esler MD, Goldstein DS, Kopin IJ: Neuronal uptake, metabolism and release of tritium-labeled norepinephrine during assessment of its plasma kinetics. Am J Physiol 1991;261: E505–E515.
8   Hoffman B, Blaschke TF, Ford GA: Beta-adrenergically mediated cardiac chronotropic and vascular smooth muscle responses during propranalol therapy and withdrawal in young and elderly persons. J Gerontol 1992;46:M22–M26.
9   Esler MD, Turner AG, Kaye DM, Thompson JM, Kingwell BA, Morris M, Lambert GW, Jennings GL, Cox HS, Seals DR: Aging effects on human sympathetic neural function. Am J Physiol 1995;268:R278–R285.
10 Van Brummelen P, Buhler FR, Kiowski W: Age-related decrease in cardiac and peripheral vascular responses to isoproterenol: Studies in normal subjects. Clin Sci 1981;60:571–577.

11   Gribbin B, Linares OA, Pickering TG, Sleight P, Pete R: Effect of age and high blood pressure on baroreflex sensitivity in man. Circ Res 1971;29:424–431.

12   Shimada K, Kitazumi T, Sadakane N, Ogura H, Ozawa T: Age related changes in baroreflex function, plasma norepinephrine and blood pressure. Hypertension 1985;7:113–117.

13   Sowers JR, Mohanty PK: Effects of advancing age on cardiopulmonary baroreceptor function in hypertensive men. Hypertension 1987;10:274–279.

14   Sowers JR, Mohanty PK: Norepinephrine and forearm vascular resistance response to tilt and cold pressor test in essential hypertension: Effects of aging. Angiology 1989;40:872–879.

15   Jeske I, Morrison SF, Cravo SL, Reis DJ: Identification of baroreceptor reflex interneurons in the caudal ventrolateral medulla. Am J Physiol 1993;264:R169–R178.

16   Sowers JR, Whitfield LA, Catania RA, Stern N, Tuck ML, Dornfeld L, Maxwell M: Role of the sympathetic nervous system in blood pressure maintenance in obesity. J Clin Endocrinol Metab 1982;54:1181–1186.

17   Daly PA, Landsberg L: Hypertension in obesity and NIDDM. Role of insulin and sympathetic nervous system. Diabetes Care 1991;14:240–248.

18   Reaven GM, Lithell H, Landsberg L: Hypertension and associated metabolic abnormalities – The role of insulin resistance and the sympathoadrenal system. N Engl J Med 1996;334:374–381.

19   Rowe JW, Troen BR: Sympathetic nervous system and aging in man. Endocr Rev 1980;1:167–179.

20   Sowers JR, Rubenstein L, Stern N: Plasma norepinephrine responses to posture and isometric exercises with age in the absence of obesity. J Gerontol 1983;38:315–317.

21   Prinz PN, Halter JB, Benedetti C, Raskind M: Circadian variation of plasma catecholamines in young and old men: Relation to rapid eye movement and slow wave sleep. J Clin Endocrinol Metab 1979;49:300–304.

22   Esler M, Skews H, Leonard P, Jackman G, Bobik A, Korner P: Age-dependence of adrenaline kinetics in normal subjects. Clin Sci 1981;60:217–219.

23   Verth RC, Featherstone JA, Linares OA, Halter JB: Age differences in plasma norepinephrine kinetics in humans. J Gerontol 1986;41:319–324.

24   Sundlof G, Wallen BG: Human muscle nerve sympathetic activity at rest: Relationship to blood pressure and age. J Physiol 1978;274:621–637.

25   Feldman RD, Limbird LE, Nadeau J, Robertson D, Wood AJ: Alterations in leukocyte beta-receptor affinity with aging: A potential explanation for altered beta-adrenergic sensitivity in the elderly. N Engl J Med 1984;310:815–819.

26   Ward KD, Sparrow D, Landsberg L, Young JB, Vokonas PS, Weiss ST: Influence of insulin, sympathetic nervous system activity, and obesity on blood pressure: The Normative Aging Study. J Hypertens 1996;14:301–308.

27   Cerasola G, Cottone S, D'Ignoto G, Grasso L, Carone MB: Sympathetic activity in borderline and established hypertension in the elderly. J Hypertens 1988;6:S55–S58.

28   Haynes WG, Sivitz WI, Morgan DA, Walsh SA, Mark AL: Sympathetic and cardiorenal actions of leptin. Hypertension 1997;30:619–623.

29   Haynes WG, Morgan DA, Walsh SA, Mark AL, Sivitz WI: Receptor-mediated regional sympathetic nerve activation by leptin. J Clin Invest 1997;100:270–278.

30   Morley JE, Baumgartner RN, Roubenoff R, Mayer J, Nair KS: Sarcopenia. J Lab Clin Med 2001; 137:231–243.

31   Fukagawa NK, Bandini LG, Young JB: Effect of age on body composition and resting metabolic rate. Am J Physiol 1990;259:E233–E238.

32   Poehlman ET, Toth MJ, Bunyard LB, Gardner AW, Donaldson KE, Colman E, Fonong T, Ades PA: Physiological predictions of increasing total and central adiposity in aging men and women. Arch Intern Med 1995;155:2443–2448.

33   Troisi RJ, Heinold JW, Vokonas PS, Weiss ST: Cigarette smoking, dietary intake, and physical activity: Effects on body fat distribution: The Normative Aging Study. Am J Clin Nutr 1991;53: 1104–1111.

34   Schwaratz RS, Shuman WP, Larson V: The effect of intensive endurance exercise training on body fat distribution in young and older men. Metabolism 1991;40:545–551.

35   Kohrt WM, Obert KA, Holloszy JO: Exercise training improves fat distribution patterns in 60 to 70 year old men and women. J Gerontol 1992;47:99–105.

36   Sowers JR: Metabolic and cardiovascular factors contributing to hypertension in the elderly; in Morley JE, van den Berg C (eds): Contemporary Endocrinology: Endocrinology of Aging. Totowa, Humana Press, 2000, pp 249–261.
37   Sowers JR, Farrow SL: Treatment of elderly hypertensive patients with diabetes, renal disease and coronary heart disease. Am J Geriatr Cardiol 1996;5:57–70.
38   Applegate WB, Sowers JR: Elevated systolic blood pressure: Increased cardiovascular risk and rationale for treatment. Am J Med 1996;101(3A):3S–9S.
39   Ali SS, Sowers JR: Update on the management of hypertension. Treatment of the elderly and diabetic hypertensives. Is the approach to management really different? Cardiovasc Res Rep 1998; 6:44–54.
40   Khoury S, Yarows SA, O'Brien TK, Sowers JR: Ambulatory blood pressure monitoring in a nonacademic setting. Effects of age and sex. Am J Hypertens 1992;5:616–623.
41   Stern N, McGinty D, Eggena P, Sowers JR: Disassociation of 24 hour calecholamine levels from blood pressure in older men. Hypertension 1985;7:1023–1029.

Prof. James R. Sowers, MD, FACE, FACP,
University of Missouri-Columbia,
Department of Internal Medicine,
MA410, Health Sciences Center,
One Hospital Drive, DCO43.00, Columbia MO 65212 (USA)
Tel. +1 573 884 2013, Fax +1 573 884 1996, E-Mail jsowers@health.missouri.edu

Kuchel GA, Hof PR (eds): Autonomic Nervous System in Old Age.
Interdiscipl Top Gerontol. Basel, Karger, 2004, vol 33, pp 53–66

....

Aging, Carbohydrate Metabolism and the Autonomic Nervous System

Kenneth M. Madden, Graydon S. Meneilly

Department of Geriatric Medicine, University of British Columbia,
Vancouver, B.C., Canada

Diseases of impaired carbohydrate metabolism, like diabetes mellitus, are highly prevalent in the aged population [1]. This has stimulated interest in how interactions between aging, carbohydrate metabolism and the autonomic nervous system contribute to impaired glucose tolerance in the older population. A documented upregulation of the adrenergic response with aging has suggested that the increased counter-regulatory influence of the sympathetic response may explain changes in carbohydrate handling in the elderly. This review will examine the changes in glucose homeostasis that occur with aging, and how the upregulation of the adrenergic response relates to these changes. In addition, the effect of aging on the adrenergic response to hypoglycemia and acute ingestion of carbohydrates will be explored.

Effect of Aging on Carbohydrate Metabolism

It has long been noted that an increase in a person's age is associated with progressive glucose intolerance [1]. Early studies involving unselected subjects found major age-related changes in glucose metabolism. Several years ago, it was recognized that age-related diseases may have had a role to play in the dramatic age-associated alteration in carbohydrate metabolism. Subsequently, investigators studied glucose metabolism in carefully selected healthy elderly subjects free from underlying disease. These investigators reported more modest changes in carbohydrate metabolism. Whether these changes were due to the process of aging itself, or due to a host of other age-associated lifestyle factors (such as increased obesity, lower physical activity, and poorer diet) is still a subject of debate. Aging has been shown to be strongly correlated with an increase in percent adipose tissue, body mass index, skinfold thickness and waist-to-hip ratio, and a decrease in $VO_{2,max}$ [2]. Changes in all of these parameters have been associated with alterations in glucose metabolism in younger patient populations. Recently, investigators have looked for evidence of a purely age-associated decline in the metabolism of carbohydrates by studying fasting blood glucose levels, glycosylated hemoglobin, and oral glucose tolerance in healthy elderly subjects who have been carefully characterized in regard to the lifestyle factors noted above.

In these elderly subjects, it has been reported that there is an age-associated rise in fasting blood glucose of approximately 1 mg/dl [3] per decade. An elevation in the proportion of glycosylated hemoglobin concentration of approximately 0.11–0.15% per year [4] has been reported by some authors, but other studies have shown a more modest effect of age once adjustments are made for measures of obesity [5]. Finally, numerous studies have examined the correlation between changes in oral glucose tolerance and aging. Large studies in carefully selected subjects have found that normal aging is associated with a modest but progressive impairment in oral glucose tolerance when other confounding variables are considered [2, 6]. In summary, the bulk of the evidence suggests that normal aging is characterized by a modest but progressive impairment in glucose tolerance. Unfortunately, the methods described above do not indicate the mechanisms underlying the age-related changes in glucose tolerance. This has led to the development of newer experimental techniques that allow researchers to examine directly the processes that control plasma glucose in both elderly and young populations.

Potential Mechanisms to Explain Impaired Carbohydrate Metabolism with Aging

Numerous mechanisms have been postulated to explain the aging-associated impairment in carbohydrate metabolism. Using variants of the glucose clamp technique, investigators have examined the effect of aging on hepatic production of glucose, insulin secretion, insulin-mediated glucose disposal, and non-insulin-mediated glucose uptake (fig. 1). The role of lifestyle factors in the age-related changes has also been carefully assessed (table 1).

Although basal hepatic glucose production is unchanged with age, hepatic glucose output is suppressed more slowly in an aged population, in response to an oral glucose challenge [7]. Basal insulin levels have been found to be both normal and increased in aged subjects [8, 9]. Hyperglycemic clamp studies have found no age effect on the overall insulin responses to glucose [9], except at very high glucose levels, suggesting that under normal conditions insulin

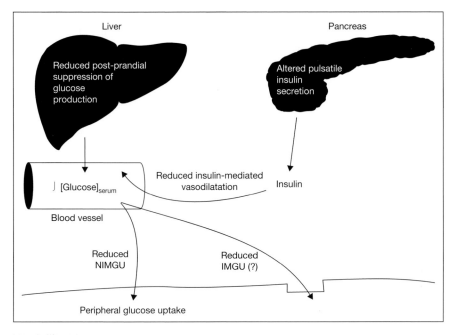

Fig. 1. This figure shows the various mechanisms by which the various components of carbohydrate metabolism (hepatic glucose production, insulin secretion, insulin-mediated glucose uptake, and non-insulin-mediated glucose uptake) interact with the normal aging process.

Table 1. Possible sites of aging-related changes in carbohydrate metabolism

---

1. Reduced hepatic production

2. Impaired insulin secretion

3. Insulin receptor (insulin-mediated glucose uptake)
   Reduction in receptor number/receptor defect
   (decreased sensitivity)
   Postreceptor defect (decreased responsiveness)

4. Impaired peripheral uptake of glucose
   (non-insulin-mediated glucose uptake)
   Change in body composition
   Impaired blood flow to skeletal muscle

5. Confounding factors
   Diet
   Degree of physical exercise
   Presence of disease

---

responses to a glucose load are unaltered. However, there appear to be more subtle alterations in insulin release with age. Several groups have demonstrated that the pulsatile production of insulin is altered with normal aging, both during fasting [10, 11] and in response to hyperglycemia [11].

It has been hypothesized that aging results in a decreased ability of insulin to stimulate glucose uptake into cells [8]. Numerous studies have evaluated insulin-mediated glucose disposal in the elderly. Although most studies have found a decline in insulin-mediated glucose uptake with age, it has been difficult to demonstrate a reduction in insulin-mediated glucose uptake with normal aging once potential confounding factors including diet, body composition and physical activity are taken into account. Two large studies examined insulin-mediated glucose uptake in carefully characterized elderly subjects. Elahi et al. [12] performed glucose clamp studies on subjects from the Baltimore longitudinal study of aging and found a modest decline in insulin-mediated glucose uptake with age. The European Group of the Study of Insulin Resistance (EGIR) demonstrated decreased insulin sensitivity during hyperinsulinemic euglycemic clamp studies of 1,146 subjects aged 18–85 but this was not significant once adjustments were made for body mass index [13]. Thus, it is uncertain whether normal aging has an effect on insulin-mediated glucose disposal.

In addition to stimulating glucose uptake, insulin also acts as a vasodilator and increases muscle blood flow. Although it is not certain whether normal aging is associated with resistance to insulin-mediated glucose uptake, the elderly clearly have a reduced vasodilatory response to insulin [14]. This could result in less blood flow to skeletal muscle, which is the primary glucose sink for the body. The potential importance of alterations in insulin-mediated blood flow in the age-related changes in glucose metabolism have yet to be determined.

Other than as indirectly affected by insulin secretion or resistance, it has been suggested that there may be an age-related change in the ability of glucose to stimulate its own uptake in the absence of insulin, otherwise known as non-insulin-mediated glucose disposal. During fasting, most non-insulin-mediated glucose uptake occurs in the central nervous system. A greater proportion of non-insulin-mediated glucose uptake occurs in muscle, splanchnic organs and adipose tissue during hyperglycemia. Studies suggest that normal aging is associated with alterations in non-insulin-mediated glucose uptake during fasting but not hyperglycemia, implying a decrease in central nervous system glucose uptake with age [15].

In summary, it appears that the glucose intolerance of aging is caused by subtle alterations in insulin secretion, altered postprandial regulation of hepatic glucose production and impaired non-insulin-mediated glucose uptake. The role of alterations in insulin-mediated glucose uptake in the glucose intolerance of aging remains uncertain.

Age-Related Changes of the Autonomic Nervous System – A Possible Explanation?

Given its diverse effects on carbohydrate metabolism [16], many researchers have turned to the autonomic nervous system as a possible explanation for these age-related changes in carbohydrate metabolism. The catecholamine response to stress acts through norepinephrine (which stimulates α- and β_1-receptors) and epinephrine (which stimulates all α- and β-receptors). As we age, a process of adrenergic upregulation occurs. This causes sympathetic neural norepinephrine release and basal levels of norepinephrine to increase with age [17]. Young et al. [18] and Blandini et al. [19] showed that basal levels of norepinephrine are increased in an aged population, while epinephrine and dopamine levels are unchanged. As well, the norepinephrine response to tilt table testing [18, 19], cold pressor test, and insulin tolerance test is also increased in an elderly population [19]. Given that the adrenergic response can act in a counter-regulatory fashion to glucose metabolism, this increased sympathetic responsiveness might explain impaired carbohydrate tolerance in the elderly.

Stress-Induced Hyperglycemia in the Aged Population

A hyperglycemic response to stress-induced sympathetic activation has been frequently documented [16]. Small doses of epinephrine similar to those observed during mild viral illness (75–80 pg/ml) given in the laboratory were shown to increase serum levels of glucose by 1.65–3.30 mmol/l in normal young subjects [20]. It seems logical, therefore that the increased sympathetic responsiveness shown in the elderly population may be a cause of elevations in blood glucose seen in a variety of clinical conditions. For example, stress-induced hyperglycemia has been documented in elderly patients in a poststroke setting [21, 22].

However, it is unclear whether age-related changes in the autonomic nervous system play a role in the day-to-day alterations in glucose metabolism which occur in the elderly. A study by Chen et al. [23] found that the basal level of norepinephrine, as well as the increase in norepinephrine with an oral glucose load did not correlate at all with glucose tolerance in both young and old subjects. This study, however, did not show an enhanced norepinephrine response to a glucose load with increasing age, which is inconsistent with the known increased adrenergic response in the elderly to other stimuli (tilt table, mental stress, cold pressor test) [18, 19] and with studies that have shown an enhanced adrenergic response to a glucose load in the elderly [18, 24]. Since no enhanced stress response was elicited by Chen et al. [23], it is difficult to argue that age-associated adrenergic hyperreactivity has no impact on glucose tolerance. Perhaps other gastrointestinal factors, such as an age-associated reduction in motility or absorption resulted in the elderly subjects receiving an effectively reduced post-prandial stimulus. An enhanced post-prandial catecholamine response still remains a possible explanation for impaired glucose metabolism in the elderly.

Aging and the Autonomic Response to Carbohydrate Intake

Investigators have tried to examine the relationship between aging-associated adrenergic changes and carbohydrate metabolism by examining the adrenergic response to acute and chronic carbohydrate ingestion. An acute oral carbohydrate load has been shown to result in an increase in norepinephrine levels in young and older subjects [18, 23]. Interestingly, Chen et al. [23] also demonstrated that there is a drop in epinephrine with an acute oral glucose load in both young and old subjects, indicating that one cannot always assume that the adrenal and the sympathetic nervous components of the adrenergic response operate in the same fashion. It has been suggested that the adrenergic response is purely due to gastrointestinal stimulation [25]. However, when the acute oral glucose response was compared with the response to an oral control drink, there was a significantly larger increase seen in norepinephrine levels in the older subjects [18, 24]. Given the effects of the sympathetic nervous system on carbohydrate metabolism discussed above, an enhanced postprandial adrenergic response is an ideal potential mechanism to explain impaired carbohydrate tolerance in the elderly.

With this in mind, Chen et al. [23] attempted to influence the adrenergic response to an oral carbohydrate load by imposing 3-day high and low carbohydrate diets. Both young and older (mean age 69) normal, screened subjects were given 3 days of a low (20–30% carbohydrate) and a high (85% carbohydrate) diet. Although the higher ingestion of carbohydrates resulted in an improved glucose tolerance, there was no effect of diet on the norepinephrine and epinephrine responses to an oral glucose load. If an increased sympathetic nervous system response to oral carbohydrate ingestion is responsible for impaired glucose tolerance in the elderly, these responses are unchanged by alterations in dietary carbohydrates in the short term [23].

Aging, Adrenergic Stimulation and Glucose Production

It has been shown previously in young normal subjects that an infusion of epinephrine results in an increase in glucose production, mostly by the liver [26, 27]. If insulin production is suppressed by somatostatin, it has been show that α-stimulation (epinephrine plus propranolol) does not increase hepatic production of glucose, indicating that sympathetic stimulation effects an increase in glucose production via the β-receptors [28]. Hepatic vein catheterization studies during radiolabeled alanine infusions on normal young humans have indicated that this β-adrenergic effect on glucose production is mediated primarily by an acute increase in glycogenolysis followed by a long-term increase in gluconeogenesis [29]. With respect to adipose tissue sources of glucose, recent work in young dogs has also shown that there is a β-adrenergic-mediated oscillatory component to lipolysis that is attenuated by β_3-blockade [30].

In aging humans, reduced sympathetic sensitivity (and consequent adrenergic upregulation) has been demonstrated throughout most of the body, but the relationship between the sympathetic nervous system and hepatic glucose production has only been investigated in aging rats [31, 32]. A study of untrained Fischer 344 rats showed that the increase in hepatic gluconeogenesis (by radiolabeled techniques) by norepinephrine infusion was attenuated by aging [31]. This attenuation may be partly explained by an uncoupling of the β-receptor and the production of adenylate cyclase production seen in isolated rat livers. Indeed, there was an observed three-fold increase in β-receptor binding capacity in the aged rat group, indicating that the change is a post-receptor phenomenon [32].

Despite this age-associated reduction in liver norepinephrine sensitivity (at a post β-receptor level), Watters et al. [33] have shown that endogenous glucose production in trauma patients actually increases with age. Although norepinephrine was not measured in this study, it is well known that the norepinephrine response is enhanced in the elderly. This suggests that the age-associated increase in the stress response was large enough to compensate for the opposing age-associated reduction in the norepinephrine sensitivity of the liver. Since there is also an enhanced norepinephrine response to a glucose load [18, 24] in elderly subjects, perhaps a similar overwhelming of attenuated liver sensitivity by an increased norepinephrine response could explain the abnormal postprandial hepatic glucose production seen in aged normal subjects [7].

Aging, Adrenergic Stimulation and Insulin Secretion

Insulin secretion is increased by stimulation of islet β_2-receptors [16] and α-adrenergic stimulation of pancreatic β-cells has been shown to reduce insulin secretion in response to a glucose stimulus. Supraphysiologic stimulation of α-receptors has been shown to reduce the acute insulin response in the rat [34, 35], and in normal young subjects [31]. Epinephrine has been shown to affect the insulin response at more physiologic levels with α-blockade increasing the insulin response in non-insulin-dependent diabetics [36] and low-dose epinephrine reducing the response in normal young subjects [37].

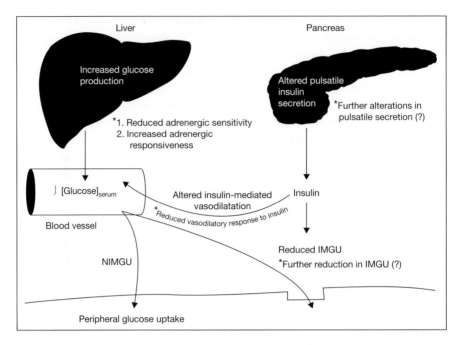

Fig. 2. This figure demonstrates various sites where the changes in carbohydrate metabolism seen in older adults are influenced by age-associated adrenergic upregulation.

Many tissues in the body, such as the heart, demonstrate a significant age-related attenuation of the response to β-receptor stimulation. It has been hypothesized that if this occurs in the pancreatic β-cell, this would result in unopposed α-stimulation (which would consequently result in reduced insulin secretion) [38]. Studies on aged rats, however, have not supported an accentuation of the effect of norepinephrine on insulin secretion in response to glucose [33]. Studies on humans aged 60+ have also failed to demonstrate an effect of aging on the effect of epinephrine on the acute insulin response to hyperglycemia [37, 38].

However, age-associated abnormalities in insulin secretion do not take the form of a simple reduction in the insulin response, but as subtle changes in pulsatile insulin secretion [10, 11, 39]. Alterations in the amplitude of low-frequency ultradian insulin pulsations have been demonstrated in pancreas transplantation (autonomically denervated) patients [40], and rapid insulin pulses are altered by electrical preganglionic nerve stimulation in the canine pancreas [41]. Although further study is required, alterations in the sympathetic nervous system are a possible explanation for the subtle age-associated changes in pulsatile insulin secretion (fig. 2).

Aging, Adrenergic Stimulation, and Insulin-Mediated Glucose Uptake

Decreased insulin sensitivity with adrenergic stimulation has been demonstrated previously in vivo in man [42]. In fact, if a somatostatin infusion is used to calculate the contribution of non-insulin-mediated glucose uptake, a 0.2 μg/kg dose of epinephrine in young subjects was found to cause a 61% decrease in insulin-mediated glucose uptake [43].

The interaction of aging with the effect of the sympathetic nervous system on insulin sensitivity is somewhat unclear. When a frequently sampled intravenous glucose tolerance test was performed on 60 human subjects aged 19–78 it was found that only body mass index and mean arterial blood pressure were significantly related to insulin sensitivity, while age, plasma norepinephrine level and epinephrine level were not [44]. In addition, the effect of small, physiologic epinephrine infusions on tolbutamide-boosted intravenous glucose tolerance tests in young and old subjects did not show any significant age-related difference in insulin action [37].

An important factor not examined in these studies is the impaired vasodilatory effect of insulin seen in the elderly [14] (fig. 2). This age-associated impairment is felt to be secondary to endothelial dysfunction, which allows the sympathetic nervous system vasoconstrictor effect to overwhelm the impaired vasodilatory effect of insulin. Given that skeletal muscle is responsible for the majority of insulin-mediated glucose disposal, this could result in reduced insulin-mediated glucose uptake. Recent studies by Meneilly et al. [45] have attempted to address this issue. Meneilly et al. showed that nitric oxide production in skeletal muscle decreases with age. However, studies involving N^G-monomethyl-L-arginine (L-NMMA) (a nitric oxide synthase inhibitor) [46] and sodium nitroprusside (a nitric oxide donor) [47] resulted in different or opposite effects on calf blood flow and insulin-mediated glucose uptake. While the combination of adrenergic upregulation (resulting in enhanced vasoconstriction) and attenuated vasodilatation by insulin may explain in part age-associated changes in insulin action, clearly much more work is needed to fully explore how aging, adrenergic upregulation, insulin action and blood flow relate.

Aging, Adrenergic Stimulation and Non-Insulin-Mediated Glucose Uptake

Rizza et al. [48] performed a study in which epinephrine was infused in the presence and absence of α- and β-blockade and in the presence and absence of insulin, glucose and glucagon. He found that epinephrine decreased glucose uptake through an undefined β-adrenergic effect on hepatic and peripheral tissues. Another study involving the administration of norepinephrine during an intravenous glucose tolerance test indicated that norepinephrine impaired the rate of glucose disposal but had no effect on 'glucose-mediated glucose disposal' (non-insulin-mediated glucose uptake) [49]. Additionally, when glucose turnover during an epinephrine infusion was measured isotopically (while somatostatin was infused to suppress pancreatic insulin secretion), it was found that epinephrine had no effect on non-insulin-mediated glucose uptake [43]. It appears that while non-insulin-mediated glucose uptake is impaired with age, this reduction is not mediated by age-associated autonomic changes. Since most non-insulin-mediated glucose uptake in the basal state occurs in the central nervous system, it is more likely that age-associated reductions in central nervous system mass are responsible for impaired non-insulin-mediated glucose uptake [15].

Effect of Aging on the Adrenergic Response to Hypoglycemia

It has been noted that the incidence of hypoglycemic complications is increased in an elderly population with diabetes [50], suggesting that perhaps there is an age-associated impairment in the counter-regulatory response to hypoglycemia. This is especially serious since it has been shown that hypoglycemia itself can cause hypoglycemia-associated autonomic failure, which can further impair the body's counter-regulatory response to (as well as symptom recognition of) hypoglycemic episodes [51]. Not only does this autonomic dysfunction impair the direct counterregulatory effects of the adrenergic system itself, it also impairs the α-cell mediated glucagon response [52] as well as the adrenergic responses to other stimuli, such as exercise [53].

In normal young subjects it has been determined that the body's primary response to hypoglycemia involves the redundant responses of both epinephrine and glucagon [54]. It has been shown that impairing the adrenergic response with the administration of clonidine will impair the early response to hypoglycemia, but not the late glucagon-mediated response [55]. Studies in young normals have shown that this response is blocked by both selective β_1- and non-selective β-blockade [56].

A study of nondiabetic elderly subjects has demonstrated an attenuated recovery from hypoglycemia induced by an intravenous dose of insulin (50 mU/kg), which was associated with a reduced glucagon response, a slightly delayed epinephrine response and no age-associated change in the norepinephrine response [57]. Meneilly et al. [58] also examined healthy young and older subjects and found that the glucose threshold for the glucagon and epinephrine response was lower in the elderly, while the norepinephrine threshold was similar between young and old (although the magnitude of the norepinephrine and epinephrine responses were similar between groups). In addition, healthy older subjects are less sensitive to the autonomic (as opposed to the neuroglycopenic) symptoms of hypoglycemia [58]. Therefore it appears that there is a mild age-associated impairment in the glucagon response, and an epinephrine response that operates at a lower threshold or is delayed. In addition, normal elderly subjects have reduced autonomic symptom awareness, possibly due to decreased end-organ sensitivity to the sympathetic nervous system response.

Conclusion

Aging is associated with an increase in fasting blood glucose, glycosylated hemoglobin and oral glucose tolerance, even after corrections are made for adiposity, diet and physical activity. This is accompanied by an age-associated process of adrenergic upregulation, in which norepinephrine levels and norepinephrine responsiveness to stimuli such as an oral glucose load increase with age. An enhanced norepinephrine response potentially explains the altered postprandial regulation of hepatic glucose production, resulting in an increase in glucose output that is not fully compensated for by an opposite age-associated reduction in liver sensitivity to norepinephrine. Aging also results in subtle changes in the pulsatile secretion of insulin, and an age-associated change in insulin action through the interaction between enhanced adrenergic-mediated vasoconstriction and attenuated insulin-mediated vasodilatation. While changes in the aging autonomic nervous system do not account for the reduction in NIMGU with age, it appears that these observed effects on hepatic glucose output, pulsatile insulin secretion, and on insulin-mediated blood flow at least partly explain the age-associated changes seen in carbohydrate metabolism. Age-associated changes in the autonomic nervous system also affect the ability of normal elderly subjects to respond to hypoglycemia. While the norepinephrine response to hypoglycemia is not impaired, the epinephrine response is delayed or operates at a lower threshold. In addition, reduced end-organ SNS sensitivity results in less awareness of the autonomic symptoms of hypoglycemia.

References

1 Harris MI: Diabetes in America: Epidemiology and scope of the problem. Diabetes Care 1998;21(suppl 3):C11–C14.
2 Shimokata H, Muller DC, Fleg JL, Sorkin J, Ziemba AW, Andres R: Age as independent determinant of glucose tolerance. Diabetes 1991;40:44–51.

3   Davidson MB: The effect of aging on carbohydrate metabolism: A review of the English literature and a practical approach to the diagnosis of diabetes mellitus in the elderly. Metabolism 1979;28:688–705.

4   Nuttall FQ: Effect of age on the percentage of hemoglobin A1c and the percentage of total glyco-hemoglobin in non-diabetic persons. J Lab Clin Med 1999;134:451–453.

5   Wiener K, Roberts NB: Age does not influence levels of HbA1c in normal subject. QJM 1999;92: 169–173.

6   Zavaroni I, Dall'Aglio E, Bruschi F, Bonora E, Alpi O, Pezzarossa A, Butturini U: Effect of age and environmental factors on glucose tolerance and insulin secretion in a worker population. J Am Geriatr Soc 1986;34:271–275.

7   Jackson RA, Hawa MI, Roshania RD, Sim BM, DiSilvio L, Jaspan JB: Influence of aging on hepatic and peripheral glucose metabolism in humans. Diabetes 1988;37:119–129.

8   Muller DC, Elahi D, Tobin JD, Andres R: The effect of age on insulin resistance and secretion: A review. Semin Nephrol 1996;16:289–298.

9   Gumbiner B, Polonsky KS, Beltz WF, Wallace P, Brechtel G, Fink RI: Effects of aging on insulin secretion. Diabetes 1989;38:1549–1556.

10 Scheen AJ, Sturis J, Polonsky KS, Van Cauter E: Alterations in the ultradian oscillations of insulin secretion and plasma glucose in aging. Diabetologia 1996;39:564–572.

11 Meneilly GS, Veldhuis JD, Elahi D: Disruption of the pulsatile and entropic modes of insulin release during an unvarying glucose stimulus in elderly individuals. J Clin Endocrinol Metab 1999;84:1938–1943.

12 Elahi D, Muller DC, McAloon-Dyke M, Tobin JD, Andres R: The effect of age on insulin response and glucose utilization during four hyperglycemic plateaus. Exp Gerontol 1993;28: 393–409.

13 Ferrannini E, Vichi S, Beck-Nielsen H, Laakso M, Paolisso G, Smith U: Insulin action and age. European Group for the Study of Insulin Resistance (EGIR). Diabetes 1996;45:947–953.

14 Meneilly GS, Elliot T, Bryer-Ash M, Floras JS: Insulin-mediated increase in blood flow is impaired in the elderly. J Clin Endocrinol Metab 1995;80:1899–1903.

15 Meneilly GS, Elahi D, Minaker KL, Sclater AL, Rowe JW: Impairment of noninsulin-mediated glucose disposal in the elderly. J Clin Endocrinol Metab 1989;68:566–571.

16 Ganong WF: Review of Medical Physiology, ed 15, rev. Norwalk, Appleton & Lange, 1995, p 330.

17 Rowe JW, Troen BR: Sympathetic nervous system and aging in man. Endocr Rev 1980; 1:167–179.

18 Young JB, Rowe JW, Pallotta JA, Sparrow D, Landsberg L: Enhanced plasma norepinephrine response to upright posture and oral glucose administration in elderly human subjects. Metabolism 1980;29:532–539.

19 Blandini F, Martignoni E, Melzi d'Eril GV, Biasio L, Sances G, Lucarelli C, Rizzo V, Costa A, Nappi G: Free plasma catecholamine levels in healthy subjects: A basal and dynamic study. The influence of age. Scand J Clin Lab Invest 1992;52:9–17.

20 Hamburg S, Hendler R, Sherwin RS: Influence of small increments of epinephrine on glucose tolerance in normal humans. Ann Intern Med 1980;93:566–568.

21 Melamed E: Reactive hyperglycaemia in patients with acute stroke. J Neurol Sci 1976;29: 267–275.

22 O'Neill PA, Davies I, Fullerton KJ, Bennett D: Stress hormone and blood glucose response following acute stroke in the elderly. Stroke 1991;22:842–847.

23 Chen M, Halter JB, Porte D Jr: Plasma catecholamines, dietary carbohydrate, and glucose intolerance: A comparison between young and old men. J Clin Endocrinol Metab 1986;62:1193–1198.

24 Tonino RP, Minaker KL, Young JB, Landsberg L, Rowe JW: Splanchnic factors enhance the norepinephrine response to oral glucose in aged man. Exp Gerontol 1986;21:413–422.

25 Tse TF, Clutter WE, Shah SD, Miller JP, Cryer PE: Neuroendocrine responses to glucose ingestion in man. Specificity, temporal relationships, and quantitative aspects. J Clin Invest 1983;72: 270–277.

26 Rizza RA, Haymond MW, Miles JM, Verdonk CA, Cryer PE, Gerich JE. Effect of alpha-adrenergic stimulation and its blockade on glucose turnover in man. Am J Physiol 1980;238: E467–E472.

27 Rizza RA, Cryer PE, Haymond MW, Gerich JE: Adrenergic mechanisms of catecholamine action on glucose homeostasis in man. Metabolism 1980;29:1155–1163.

28 Best JD, Ward WK, Pfeifer MA, Halter JB: Lack of a direct alpha-adrenergic effect of epinephrine on glucose production in human subjects. Am J Physiol 1984;246:E271–E276.

29 Sacca L, Vigorito C, Cicala M, Corso G, Sherwin RS: Role of gluconeogenesis in epinephrine-stimulated hepatic glucose production in humans. Am J Physiol 1983;245:E294–E302.

30 Hucking K, Hamilton-Wessler M, Ellmerer M, Bergman RN: Burst-like control of lipolysis by the sympathetic nervous system in vivo. J Clin Invest 2003;111:257–264.

31 Podolin DA, Gleeson TT, Mazzeo RS: Role of norepinephrine in hepatic gluconeogenesis: Evidence of aging and training effects. Am J Physiol 1994;267:E680–E686.

32 Dax EM, Partilla JS, Pineyro MA, Gregerman RI: Beta-adrenergic receptors, glucagon receptors, and their relationship to adenylate cyclase in rat liver during aging. Endocrinology 1987;120: 1534–1541.

33 Watters JM, Norris SB, Kirkpatrick SM: Endogenous glucose production following injury increases with age. J Clin Endocrinol Metab 1997;82:3005–3010.

34 McDonald RB, Herrmann S, Curry DL: Norepinephrine sensitivity of the endocrine pancreas in aging F344 rats. Aging (Milano) 1992;4:227–230.

35 Reaven E, Wright D, Mondon CE, Solomon R, Ho H, Reaven GM: Effect of age and diet on insulin secretion and insulin action in the rat. Diabetes 1983;32:175–180.

36 Broadstone VL, Pfeifer MA, Bajaj V, Stagner JI, Samols E: Alpha-adrenergic blockade improves glucose-potentiated insulin secretion in non-insulin-dependent diabetes mellitus. Diabetes 1987; 36:932–937.

37 Morrow LA, Morganroth GS, Herman WH, Bergman RN, Halter JB: Effects of epinephrine on insulin secretion and action in humans. Interaction with aging. Diabetes 1993;42:307–315.

38 Morrow LA, Rosen SG, Halter JB: Beta-adrenergic regulation of insulin secretion: Evidence of tissue heterogeneity of beta-adrenergic responsiveness in the elderly. J Gerontol 1991;46: M108–M113.

39 Meneilly GS, Ryan AS, Veldhuis JD, Elahi D: Increased disorderliness of basal insulin release, attenuated insulin secretory burst mass, and reduced ultradian rhythmicity of insulin secretion in older individuals. J Clin Endocrinol Metab 1997;82:4088–4093.

40 Sonnenberg GE, Hoffmann RG, Johnson CP, Kissebah AH: Low- and high-frequency insulin secretion pulses in normal subjects and pancreas transplant recipients: Role of extrinsic innervation. J Clin Invest 1992;90:545–553.

41 Sha L, Westerlund J, Szurszewski JH, Bergsten P: Amplitude modulation of pulsatile insulin secretion by intrapancreatic ganglion neurons. Diabetes 2001;50:51–55.

42 Robertson RP, Porte D Jr: Adrenergic modulation of basal insulin secretion in man. Diabetes 1973;22:1–8.

43 Baron AD, Wallace P, Olefsky JM: In vivo regulation of non-insulin-mediated and insulin-mediated glucose uptake by epinephrine. J Clin Endocrinol Metab 1987;64:889–895.

44 Supiano MA, Hogikyan RV, Morrow LA, Ortiz-Alonso FJ, Herman WH, Galecki AT, Halter JB: Aging and insulin sensitivity: Role of blood pressure and sympathetic nervous system activity. J Gerontol 1993;48:M237–M243.

45 Meneilly GS, Elliott T, Battistini B, Floras JS: N^G-monomethyl-L-arginine alters insulin-mediated calf blood flow but not glucose disposal in the elderly. Metabolism 2001;50:306–310.

46 Meneilly GS, Battistini B, Floras JS: Contrasting effects of L-arginine on insulin-mediated blood flow and glucose disposal in the elderly. Metabolism 2001;50:194–199.

47 Meneilly GS, Battistini B, Floras JS: Lack of effect of sodium nitroprusside on insulin-mediated blood flow and glucose disposal in the elderly. Metabolism 2000;49:373–378.

48 Rizza RA, Cryer PE, Haymond MW, Gerich JE: Adrenergic mechanisms for the effects of epinephrine on glucose production and clearance in man. J Clin Invest 1980;65:682–689.

49 Marangou AG, Alford FP, Ward G, Liskaser F, Aitken PM, Weber KM, Boston RC, Best JD: Hormonal effects of norepinephrine on acute glucose disposal in humans: A minimal model analysis. Metabolism 1988;37:885–891.

50 Morley JE: The elderly type 2 diabetic patient: Special considerations. Diabet Med 1998;15: S41–S46.

51   Dagogo-Jack SE, Craft S, Cryer PE: Hypoglycemia-associated autonomic failure in insulin-dependent diabetes mellitus. Recent antecedent hypoglycemia reduces autonomic responses to, symptoms of, and defense against subsequent hypoglycemia. J Clin Invest 1993;91:819–828.

52   Taborsky GJ Jr, Ahren B, Havel PJ: Autonomic mediation of glucagon secretion during hypoglycemia: Implications for impaired alpha-cell responses in type 1 diabetes. Diabetes 1998;47:995–1005.

53   Davis SN, Galassetti P, Wasserman DH, Tate D: Effects of antecedent hypoglycemia on subsequent counterregulatory responses to exercise. Diabetes 2000;49:73–81.

54   Cryer PE, Tse TF, Clutter WE, Shah SD: Roles of glucagon and epinephrine in hypoglycemic and nonhypoglycemic glucose counterregulation in humans. Am J Physiol 1984;247:E198–E205.

55   Metz SA, Halter JB: Effects of clonidine on hormone and substrate responses to hypoglycemia. Clin Pharmacol Ther 1980;28:441–448.

56   Popp DA, Tse TF, Shah SD, Clutter WE, Cryer PE: Oral propranolol and metoprolol both impair glucose recovery from insulin-induced hypoglycemia in insulin-dependent diabetes mellitus. Diabetes Care 1984;7:243–247.

57   Marker JC, Cryer PE, Clutter WE: Attenuated glucose recovery from hypoglycemia in the elderly. Diabetes 1992;41:671–678.

58   Meneilly GS, Cheung E, Tuokko H: Altered responses to hypoglycemia of healthy elderly people. J Clin Endocrinol Metab 1994;78:1341–1348.

Dr. Kenneth M. Madden
Department of Geriatric Medicine
University of British Columbia, Vancouver, B.C. (Canada)
Tel. +1 604 822 0750, Fax +1 604 822 0755, E-Mail kmmadden@interchange.ubc.ca

Kuchel GA, Hof PR (eds): Autonomic Nervous System in Old Age.
Interdiscipl Top Gerontol. Basel, Karger, 2004, vol 33, pp 67–77

··················

Aging and the Gastrointestinal Tract

Alberto Pilotto[a], *Marilisa Franceschi*[b], *Giuseppe Orsitto*[a],
Leandro Cascavilla[a]

[a]UO Geriatrics, IRCCS Casa Sollievo della Sofferenza,
San Giovanni Rotondo, and [b]UO Geriatrics, Schio Hospital, Schio (VI), Italy

The Aging Esophagus

The term 'presbyesophagus' was used to describe a spectrum of changes affecting the esophagus in old age, including decreased contractile amplitude, polyphasic waves in the esophageal body, incomplete sphincter relaxation and esophageal dilatation. More recently, investigators using modern techniques and classification systems, have challenged this concept [1]. In fact, recent manometric studies have demonstrated the presence of only minor alterations in esophageal motility in healthy elderly subjects [2]. Additional studies have reported other age-related changes, including a decrease in upper esophageal sphincter (UES) pressure [3] with a deterioration of the pharyngo-UES contractile reflex [4]. During swallowing, the timing of the pressure fall at the UES was significantly delayed in the elderly when compared to young subjects, with the UES pressure reaching its minimum value after the arrival of the bolus at the UES [5]. In agreement with these findings, a delay in relaxation after deglution [6] and a reduction of the secondary esophageal peristalsis evoked by esophageal distension were also reported in the elderly [7]. Such changes in swallowing pressures and laryngeal movements with aging may have an impact on the system which normally prevents aspiration, thus explaining the high prevalence of dysphagia in old age.

A recent manometric study conducted in 79 healthy subjects reported that age correlated inversely with the pressure and length of the lower esophageal sphincter (LES), while simultaneous contraction appeared to increase with age [8]. These results are in agreement with a previous finding demonstrating an increase in the prevalence of tertiary contractions [9], which together with a failure of esophageal contraction after swallowing, contributes to incomplete esophageal emptying of both low- and high-viscosity liquids seen in elderly subjects [10]. Moreover, a manometric and scintigraphic study of healthy volunteers aged 20–80 years documented that older persons have more frequently abnormal peristalsis and a longer duration of gastroesophageal reflux episodes than young or middle-aged subjects [11]. These findings may explain the higher severity of reflux esophagitis in older people [12].

The morphological origin of such functional alterations is not well established. Although the thickness of the human esophageal smooth muscle does not vary with aging [13], the numbers of myenteric neurons in the esophagus decline with age [14], the decrease being most pronounced in the proximal esophagus, particularly at its junction with the pharynx [14].

The clinical significance of these findings is also unclear. Many of the above studies failed to show a clear correlation between modifications in esophageal function and symptomatology, particularly dysphagia [3, 9, 10]. One important consideration is that the currently used 'normal values' for parameters of esophageal function may change with age. As a result, these parameters, may not be directly comparable in young and old subjects. For example, a radiologic study performed in elderly asymptomatic subjects found that only 16% had swallowing within the normal limits as defined in younger subjects [15]. Moreover, a study of 24-hour esophageal pH monitoring demonstrated that 30% of asymptomatic elderly subjects were 'abnormal' according to conventional 24-hour pH-metric criteria [16]. With these considerations in mind, it has been proposed that 'age-related normality limits' of esophageal pressures need to be considered before establishing a manometric diagnosis in elderly patients [8]. Thus, the current view of esophageal dysfunction which has been derived from studies involving younger subjects may need to be modified before being applied to the geriatric age group.

Particular attention has been given to the clinical presentation of gastroesophageal reflux disease (GERD) in the elderly, since important differences appear to exist in the symptomatology involving young as compared to adult patients [17]. An age-related decline in the sensitivity of esophageal to visceral pain has been documented by studies using esophageal balloon distension [18]. These findings combined with a reduction in esophageal chemosensitivity to acid with advancing age [19] may explain such different clinical expression of GERD in patients of different ages. However, other factors may also be involved in GERD presenting in the elderly. These may be secondary to systemic diseases, with contributions due to decreased salivary secretion, alterations in gastric emptying, decreased tissue resistance as a result of impaired epithelial cell regeneration, or a duodenogastro-esophageal reflux of bile salts [20].

In conclusion, declines in esophageal function do not appear to be an inevitable consequence of aging, yet the esophagus does undergo specific changes with aging. These changes need to be taken into account in the evaluation of older patients with esophageal complaints [1].

The Aging Stomach

Aggressive Factors

A progressive reduction in gastric acid secretion is believed to occur with increasing age, principally due to atrophy of gastric mucosa. In 1982, Kekki et al. [21] demonstrated that gastric acid secretion did not change with age in the absence of chronic atrophic gastritis and, successively, several studies demonstrated that gastric acid secretion did not change in normal elderly subjects [22, 23], declining only in the presence of coexisting gastric pathology related to *Helicobacter pylori* infection [24]. A more recent study confirmed that advancing age had no independent effect on gastric acid secretion [25] and a study performed in 427 peptic ulcer patients showed no significant differences in the various age groups in terms of basal and pentagastrin-stimulated acid secretion [26].

Recent studies have explored the role of *H. pylori* infection on gastric acid secretion in relation to age. A Japanese group had reported that both basal and maximal acid output decreased with age in *H. pylori*-positive subjects, while they did not change with age in *H. pylori*-negative subjects [27]; moreover, the study confirmed that gastric acid secretion decreased with the progression of atrophic gastritis and that the development of such atrophic changes of the gastric mucosa were more closely related to *H. pylori* infection than to age [28]. The significant association between gastric atrophy and the presence of Cag-A positive strains of *H. pylori* in the gastric mucosa of elderly subjects [29], as well as the recent finding that *H. pylori* eradication is beneficial in preventing progression of gastric atrophy in patients >45 years old [30], corroborates the hypothesis that *H. pylori* infection may be more a important factor in inducing gastric mucosa modifications than aging.

Conflicting data are present in the literature regarding pepsin secretion in old age. Levels of serum pepsinogen A (or group I, PGA) were unchanged in older *H. pylori*-negative subjects, indicating that the release of pepsin from chief and mucous neck cells appears to be maintained in these individuals. In contrast, older patients with *H. pylori* infection, exhibited higher levels of PGA and pepsinogen C (or group II, PGC), with a decrease in the PGA/PGC ratio [31]. Interestingly, the eradication of *H. pylori* from the stomach of older patients induced a rapid and significant decrease in PGC, together with an increase in the PGA/PGC ratio [31].

In conclusion, available data support the notion that aging by itself does not modify gastric aggressive factors, such as acid and pepsin secretions. Moreover, pathological conditions, principally *H. pylori* infection, may induce some mucosal alterations (chronic gastritis, gastric atrophy and intestinal metaplasia) that may influence some changes in gastric secretory functions. The temporal sequence of these pathogenetic events remains unknown, yet it appears unlikely that this disease process would remain reversible in its latter stages.

Defensive Factors

Many factors contribute to the ability of the gastric mucosal barrier to resist external damage, including an adherent mucus gel, prostaglandin and bicarbonate secretions, gastric mucosal proliferation and gastric mucosal blood flow. Interestingly, recent studies indicate that many of these aspects of the gastric mucosal barrier could change in old age. Clinical studies have demonstrated that gastric mucosal prostaglandin concentrations decline with age [32, 33]. Similar results were obtained in animal studies, indicating that aged animals with low gastric mucosal prostaglandin levels were more susceptible to aspirin-induced acute gastric damage [34]. Gastric bicarbonate and mucus are secreted by nonparietal gastric epithelial cells, providing an alkaline gel layer protective against luminal acid-pepsin and exogenous noxious substances. Two studies have shown that aging was associated with significantly lower gastric bicarbonate secretion [35, 36] and mucus production [36] in humans. Moreover, in agreement with previous data [37], the quality of mucus secretion was unaltered with advancing age [36]. More recently, a study that examined the thickness of the adherent mucus gel layer in the gastric antrum and duodenum in relation to age, showed a significant thinning of the adherent mucus gel layer in *H. pylori*-positive individuals, as stomach and duodenum age. In those without *H. pylori* infection, the mucus gel thickness was preserved in stomach and duodenum [38].

As regards gastric mucosal proliferation, a study in healthy subjects demonstrated that the number of gastric mucus cells was reduced in the elderly, with aging having induced a significant increase in the parietal:mucous cell ratio [39]. Successively, animal studies demonstrated that aging was associated with a diminished regenerative capacity of the gastric mucosa [40], secondary to a reduced expression of several growth factors and of enzymes related to growth factor receptors [41]. The role of gastric mucosal blood flow in maintaining the gastric mucosal integrity in humans, and particularly in the elderly, is not well defined. A study in animals has shown that aging was associated with a significant decline in basal gastric blood flow, whereas no impairment occurred in acid-induced gastric blood flow [42]. More recently, a study carried out in 24 elderly patients devoid of endoscopic abnormalities and in a matching group of younger subjects reported that gastric mucosal perfusion was significantly decreased in aged subjects [36].

In conclusion, available data seem to support the concept that aging is associated with a selective and specific reduction in some gastric mucosal defensive mechanisms [43]. A better understanding of these age-related changes will aid in the development of new interventions for the prevention of gastric mucosal injury, particularly that due to the toxic effect of exogenous substances such as drugs.

Motility

It is generally agreed that motility and gastric emptying time progressively diminish with advancing age. Previous studies carried out with radium-marked solid and liquid meals have demonstrated that the vagus-mediated emptying of liquids becomes slower, while there does not seem to be any difference between the elderly and young adults as regards emptying time for solid meals [44]. In contrast, other authors have suggested that aging is associated with a general slowing in gastric emptying for both liquids and solids [45]. These studies failed to take into account the influence of gastric acid secretion on the emptying of the stomach. A manometric study demonstrated that alterations in gastric motility of elderly subjects consisted predominantly of a lower incidence of phase III activity which was unrelated to the gastric acid secretion [46]. Interestingly, motilin levels were generally elevated, while periodic plasma changes were smaller in the elderly compared to young subjects [47].

More recently, delayed gastric emptying of solid foods, evaluated by ultrasound, has been reported in elderly subjects compared to young subjects [48]. Another study, using electrical impedance tomography, demonstrated that gastric emptying of liquid meals was longer in the elderly than in the young subjects when lipids (triglycerides, 24.6 g) were included in the liquid test meals, while gastric emptying time for non-lipid soup was not significantly different between the elderly and young subjects [49]. The reasons of such motility modifications with age are not clear; however delayed gastric emptying could result from progressive autonomic nerve dysfunction occurring with aging [48]. Indeed, a recent experimental study carried out in male Fisher 344 rats reported that in the stomach, both the vagal and myenteric innervation were stable between the ages of 3 and 24 months; however, a decrease in the number of myenteric neurons in the forestomach was noted at 27 months [50]. In contrast, clinical data from patients with diabetes mellitus indicated that, even if gastroparesis and upper GI symptoms have been attributed to irreversible autonomic damage, metabolic factors such as acute changes in the blood-glucose concentration, are likely to have a major effect on gastric motor function [51].

Indeed, gastric emptying appeared to slow during hyperglycemia, accelerating with hypoglycemia [51].

An interesting recent study evaluated the effects of aging on fasting gastric compliance and the perception of gastric distension as well as the gastric accommodation to a meal [52]. The results suggested that healthy aging is associated with decreased perception of gastric distension without any change in fasting gastric compliance and with reduced tone late in the postprandial period when compared with younger individuals. Thus, the control of food intake appeared to be less sensitive to external stimuli in older than in young subjects. These data are in agreement with the observation that the early satiation observed in the elderly appears to be predominantly due to a decrease in adaptive relaxation of the fundus of the stomach resulting in early antral filling [53]. However, increased levels and effectiveness of cholecystokinin, which may contribute to the slowing of gastric emptying [54], may also play a role in the anorexia of aging. In terms of the central feeding drive, both the opioid and neuropeptide Y effects appear to decline with age [54]. It is possible that these physiologic changes associated with aging could increase the risk for older persons to develop severe anorexia and weight loss when disease occurs [53], while also contributing to gastroduodenal pathology such as peptic ulcer disease [55].

Aging and the Small Intestine

Although minor differences in morphology of the small intestine between young adult and elderly subjects including shorter villi in older subjects have been described, these observations have not been replicated by other studies [56]. Specific enzymes may decrease with age. Declines in the levels of one of these enzymes, lactase, may lead to lactose intolerance. Although lactase activity may decrease with age, human small intestine maltase and sucrase concentrations are usually preserved. The integrity of the small intestine, as assessed by its permeability, is known to be altered by a variety of diseases, such as Crohn's disease and celiac disease. Until recently, it had remained unclear whether normal aging influences small intestine integrity. The ratio of absorption of orally ingested lactulose to mannitol is used as a measure of small intestine permeability. Clinical studies have indicated that the small intestine permeability of adults aged over 60 years was similar to that of younger adults [57]. More recently, other studies reported that α_1-antitrypsin clearance, a measure of the 'leakiness' of the gut from the body into the gut lumen, was not different between older healthy subjects and younger adults [58]. Thus, small intestinal permeability or integrity does not seem to change with age.

It is difficult to measure small intestine motility clinically. Human studies have shown that small intestine transit time remained relatively stable with increasing age [48, 59]. However, using the hydrogen breath test after administration of 10 g lactulose, the orocecal transit time (OCTT) was found to be significantly longer in healthy elderly than in healthy young adult subjects [60]. Another study reported that more than 60% of elderly subjects showed abnormal breath hydrogen excretion after eating a 200-gram carbohydrate meal [56]. This breath hydrogen rise may be caused by increased bacterial metabolism of carbohydrate, either from contact within the proximal small bowel or within the colon. Thus, from these studies, it is unclear whether the elevated breath hydrogen was caused by lower OCTT or bacterial overgrowth of the small intestine [59, 60]. In fact, a number of diseases that can affect small intestine motility, such as diabetes, thyroid disorders and scleroderma, are increasingly prevalent in older age groups. In the absence of such diseases, motility seems to be unaffected by age [61].

The Aging Colon

Aging is associated with changes in the structure and function of the colon. With aging, a progressive alteration in the mechanical properties of the colonic wall has been described. This change depends, at least partially, on changes in ultrastructure. Collagens, which form a submucosal network of fibrils, become smaller and more tightly packed in the left colon with aging [62]. An accumulation of collagenous proteins has been described to occur in old rats and this was accompanied by a decrease in the tensile strength that may cause deterioration of the functional integrity of the left colonic wall [63]. It is conceivable that such ultrastructural changes may reduce the compliance of the colon with aging, and that this might play a role in the development of diverticulosis.

Control of colonic motility is complex. Indeed, several factors including extrinsic innervation, myenteric plexus neurons, neurotransmitter release, smooth muscle responsiveness and gastrointestinal hormones may influence colonic motor functions. Aging has been associated with changes in smooth muscle function. Animal studies showed that the thickness of the external smooth muscle layers of the gastrointestinal tract and the individual smooth muscle cells continue to grow in size with aging. This phenomenon is associated with an increased production of collagen by these cells, thereby altering the extracellular matrix [47]. Moreover, older colonic muscle cells respond less to a variety of stimuli including acetylcholine or electrical field stimulation, than do cells from younger adult animals [64], probably due to changes in calcium-channels that occur with aging [65]. In the ganglia of the myenteric plexus, aging is associated with a reduced number of neurons in animals [50, 66]. In humans also the total number of neurons in the myenteric plexus was decreased [67]. However, it remains unclear whether the myenteric neuronal fall-out with aging is clinically relevant or whether the redundancy of neurons (100 million in the adult mammalian gut) provides a functional reserve of surviving neurons that compensates for the neuronal loss with aging [68]. The function of the inhibitory neurons in the myenteric plexus in the human colon decreases with advancing age [69]. Such function is mediated by non-adrenergic and noncholinergic (NANC) inhibitory innervation. While colonic concentrations of NANC inhibitory neuropeptides (vasoactive intestinal peptide, peptide histidine-methionine, met-5-enkephalin, neuropeptide Y and somatostatin) were comparable in colons from older and younger subjects, recent data from animals suggest that nitrergic (nitric oxide) innervation may play a key role in the relaxation of the normal colon and that such inhibitory effect of nitric oxide innervation significantly decreased with aging [70]. The rate of this loss of nitric oxide relaxation with age in humans in unknown. Nevertheless, understanding the relative contributions of these mechanisms to colonic relaxation may lead to novel therapeutic approaches towards some very common geriatric diseases such as diverticulosis, constipation and irritable bowel syndrome [68].

References

1   De Vault KR: Presbyesophagus: A reappraisal. Curr Gastronterol Rep 2002;4:193–199.
2   Adamek RJ, Wegener M, Wienbeck M, Gielen B: Long-term oesophageal manometry in healthy subjects. Evaluation of normal values and influence of age. Dig Dis Sci 1994;39:2069–2073.
3   Shaker R, Lang IM: Effect of aging on the deglutitive oral, pharyngeal, and oesophageal motor function. Dysphagia 1994;9:221–228.
4   Ren J, Xie P, Lang IM, et al: Deterioration of the pharyngo-UES contractile reflex in the elderly. Laryngoscope 2000;110:1563–1566.
5   Yokoyama M, Mitomi N, Tetsuka K, et al: Role of laryngeal movement and effect of aging on swallowing pressure in the pharings and upper esophageal sphincter. Laryngoscope 2000;110: 434–439.
6   Fulp SR, Dalton CB, Castell JA, Castell DO: Aging-related alterations in human upper esophageal sphincter function. Am J Gastroenterol 1990;85:1569–1572.
7   Ren J, Shaker R, Kusano M, et al: Effect of aging on the secondary esophageal peristalsis: Presbyesophagus revisited. Am J Physiol 1995;268:G772–G779.
8   Grande L, Lacima G, Ros E, et al: Deterioration of esophageal motility with age: A manometric study of 79 healthy subjects. Am J Gastroenterol 1999;94:1795–1801.
9   Grishaw EK, Ott DJ, Frederick MG, et al: Functional abnormalities of the esophagus: A prospective analysis of radiographic findings relative to age and symptoms. Am J Roentgenol 1996;167: 719–723.
10   Ferriolli E, Dantas RO, Oliveira RB, Braga FJ: The influence of ageing on oesophageal motility after ingestion of liquids with different viscosities. Eur J Gastroenterol Hepatol 1996;8:793–798.
11   Ferriolli E, Oliveira RB, Matsuda NM, et al: Aging, esophageal motility, and gastroesophageal reflux. J Am Geriatr Soc 1998;46:1534–1537.

12   Collen MJ, Abdullian JD, Chen YC: Gastroesophageal reflux disease in the elderly: More severe disease that requires aggressive therapy. Am J Gastroenterol 1995;90:1053–1057.

13   Eckardt VF, Le Compte PM: Esophageal ganglia and smooth muscle in the elderly. Dig Dis Sci 1978;23:849–856.

14   Meciano-Filho J, Carvalho VC, De Souza RR: Nerve cell loss in the myenteric plexus of the human esophagus in relation to age: A preliminary investigation. Gerontology 1995;41:18–21.

15   Ekberg O, Feinberg MJ: Altered swallowing function in elderly patients without dysphagia: Radiologic findings in 56 cases. Am J Roentgenol 1991;156:1181–1184.

16   Fass R, Sampliner RE, Mackel C, et al: Age- and gender-related differences in 24-hour esophageal pH monitoring of normal subjects. Dig Dis Sci 1993;38:1926–1928.

17   Pilotto A, Di Mario F, Malfertheiner P, et al: Upper gastrointestinal diseases in the elderly. Eur J Gastroenterol Hepatol 1999;11:801–808.

18   Lasch H, Castell DO, Castell JA: Evidence for diminished visceral pain with aging: Studies using graded intraesophageal balloon distension. Am J Physiol 1997;272:G1–G3.

19   Fass R, Pulliam G, Johnson C, et al: Symptom severity and oesophageal chemosensitivity to acid in older and young patients with gastro-oesophageal reflux. Age Ageing 2000;29:125–130.

20   Tack J, VanTrappen G: The aging esophagus. Gut 1997;41:422–424.

21   Kekki M, Samloff IM, Ihamaki T, et al: Age- and sex-related behaviour of gastric acid secretion at the population level. Scand J Gastroenterol 1982;17:737–743.

22   Goldschmiedt M, Barnett CC, Schwarz BE, et al: Effect of age on gastric acid secretion and serum gastrin concentrations in healthy men and women. Gastroenterology 1991;101:977–990.

23   Collen MJ, Abdullian JD, Chen YK: Age does not affect basal gastric acid secretion in normal subjects or in patients with acid-peptic disease. Am J Gastroenterol 1994;89:712–716.

24   Katelaris PH, Seow F, Lin BPC, et al: Effect of age, Helicobacter pylori infection, and gastritis with atrophy on serum gastrin and gastric acid secretion in healthy men. Gut 1993;34:1032–1037.

25   Feldman M, Cryer B, McArthur KE, et al: Efects of aging and gastritis on gastric acid and pepsin secretion in humans: A prospective study. Gastroenterology 1996;110:1043–1052.

26   Pilotto A, Vianello F, Di Mario F, et al: Effect of age on gastric acid, pepsin, pepsinogen group A and gastrin in peptic ulcer patients. Gerontology 1994;40:253–259.

27   Haruma K, Kamada T, Kawaguchi H, et al: Effect of age and Helicobacter pylori infection on gastric acid secretion. J Gastroenterol Hepatol 2000;15:277–283.

28   Pilotto A, Malfertheiner P: An approach to Helicobacter pylori infection in the elderly. Aliment Pharmacol Ther 2002;16:683–691.

29   Pilotto A, Rassu M, Bozzola L, et al: Cag-A positive Helicobacter pylori infection in the elderly. Association with gastric atrophy and intestinal metaplasia. J Clin Gastroenterol 1998;26:18–22.

30   Sung JJ, Lin S, Ching JY, et al: Atrophy and intestinal metaplasia one year after cure of H. pylori infection: A prospective randomized study. Gastroenterology 2000;119:7–14.

31   Pilotto A, Franceschi M, Leandro G, et al: The clinical usefulness of serum pepsinogens, specific IgG anti-Hp antibodies and gastrin for monitoring Helicobacter pylori treatment in older people. J Am Geriatr Soc 1996;44:665–670.

32   Cryer B, Redfern JS, Goldschmeidt M, et al: Effect of aging on gastric and duodenal mucosal prostaglandin concentrations in humans. Gastroenterology 1992;102:1118–1123.

33   Goto H, Sugiyama S, Ohara A, et al: Age-associated decrease in prostaglandins contents in human gastric mucosa. Biochem Biophys Res Commun 1992;186:1443–1448.

34   Lee M, Feldman M: Age-related reductions in gastric mucosal prostaglandins levels increase susceptibility to aspirin-induced injury in rats. Gastroenterology 1994;107:1746–1750.

35   Feldman M, Cryer B: Effects of age on gastric alkaline and non-parietal fluid secretion in humans. Gerontology 1998;44:222–227.

36   Guslandi M, Pellegrini A, Sorghi M: Gastric mucosal defences in the elderly. Gerontology 1999; 45:206–208.

37   Pilotto A, Dal Santo PL, Di Mario F, et al: Pepsin and mucus secretion in elderly subjects affected by upper upper GI diseases. Giorn Gerontol 1988;36:265–270.

38   Newton JL, Jordan N, Pearson J, et al: The adherent gastric antral and duodenal mucus gel layer thins with advancing age in subjects infected with Helicobacter pylori. Gerontology 2000;46: 153–157.

39   Farinati F, Formentini S, Della Libera G, et al: Changes in parietal and mucous cell mass in the gastric mucosa of normal subjects with age: A morphometric study. Gerontology 1993;39: 146–151.

40   Fligiel SEG, Relan NK, Dutta S, et al: Aging diminishes gastric mucosal regeneration: Relationship to tyrosine kinases. Lab Invest 1994;70:764–774.

41   Relan NK, Fligiel SEG, Dutta S, et al: Induction of EGF-receptor tyrosine kinase during early reparative phase of gastric mucosa and effects of aging. Lab Invest 1995;73:717–726.

42   Lee M: Age-related changes in gastric blood flow in rats. Gerontology 1996;42:290–293.

43   Majumdar AP, Fligiel SE, Jaszewski R: Gastric mucosal injury and repair: Effect of aging. Histol Histopathol 1997;12:491–501.

44   Moore JG, Tweedy C, Christian PE, et al: Effect of age on gastric emptying of liquid and solid meals in man. Dig Dis Sci 1983;28:340–344.

45   Horowitz M, Maddern GJ, Chatterton BE, et al: Changes in gastric emptying rates with age. Clin Sci 1984;67:213–218.

46   Bortolotti M, Fradà G, Vezzadini P, et al: Influence of gastric acid secretion on interdigestive gastric motor activity and serum motilin in the elderly. Digestion 1987;38:226–233.

47   Szurszewski JH, Holt PR, Schuster M: Proceedings of a Workshop entitled 'Neuromuscular function and dysfunction of the gastrointestinal tract in aging'. Dig Dis Sci 1989;34:1135–1146.

48   Brogna A, Ferrara R, Bucceri AM, et al: Influence of aging on gastrointestinal transit time. An ultrasonographic and radiologic study. Invest Radiol 1999;34:357–359.

49   Nakae Y, Onouchi H, Kagaya M, Kondo T: Effects of aging and gastric lipolysis on gastric emptying of lipid in liquid meal. J Gastroenterol 1999;34:445–449.

50   Phillips RJ, Powley TL: As the gut ages: Timetables for aging of innervation vary by organ in the Fisher 344 rat. J Comp Neurol 2001;434:358–377.

51   Kong MF, Horowitz M: Gastric emptying in diabetes mellitus: Relationship to blood-glucose control. Clin Geriatr Med 1999;15:321–338.

52   Rayner CK, MacIntosh CG, Chapman IM, et al: Effects of age on proximal gastric motor and sensory function. Scand J Gastroenterol 2000;35:1041–1047.

53   Morley JE, Thomas DR: Anorexia and aging: Pathophysiology. Nutrition 1999;15:499–503.

54   MacIntosh CG, Andrews JM, Jones KL, et al: Effects of age on concentrations of plasma chole-cystokinin, glucagon-like peptide 1, and peptide YY and their relation to appetite and pyloric motility. Am J Clin Nutr 1999;69:999–1006.

55   Dal Santo PL, Germanà B, Del Bianco T: Gastroduodenal motility in the elderly; in Pilotto A, Di Mario F, Vigneri S (eds): Ulcer Disease in the Elderly. Padova, Piccin, 1996, pp 39–45.

56   Saltzman JR, Russel RM: Gastrointestinal function and aging; in Morley JE, Glick Z, Rubenstein LZ (eds): Geriatric Nutrition, ed 2. New York, Raven Press, 1995, pp 183–189.

57   Saltzman JR, Kowdley KV, Perrone G, et al: Changes in small-intestine permeability with ageing. J Am Geriatr Soc 1995;43:160–164.

58   Saltzman JR, Russel RM: The ageing gut: Nutritional issues. Gastroenterol Clin N Am 1998; 27:309–324.

59   Dal Santo PL, Chioatto P, Menegolli G, et al: Influence of ageing on oro-caecal transit time and intestinal hydrogen production. Rec Adv Aging Sci 1993;II:1097–1102.

60   Pilotto A, Franceschi M, Del Favero G, et al: The effect of aging on oro-cecal transit time in normal subjects and patients with gallstone disease. Aging Clin Exp Res 1995;7:234–237.

61   Saltzman JR, Karamitsios N: Diseases of the small intestine and pancreas; in Evans JG, Williams TF, et al (eds): Oxford Textbook of Geriatric Medicine, ed 2. Oxford, Oxford University Press, 2000, pp 285–299.

62   Thomson HJ, Busuttil A, Eastwood MA, et al: Submucosal collagen changes in the normal colon and in diverticular disease. Int J Colorect Dis 1987;2:208–213.

63   Christensen H, Andreassen TT, Oxlund H: Age-related alterations in the strength and collagen content of left colon in rats. Int J Colorect Dis 1992;7:85–88.

64   Roberts D, Gelperin D, Wiley JW: Evidence for age-associated reduction in acetylcholine release and smooth muscle response in the rat colon. Am J Physiol 1994;267:G515–G522.

65   Xiong Z, Sperelakis N, Noffsinger A, et al: Changes in calcium channel current densities in rat colonic smooth muscle cells during development and aging. Am J Physiol 1993;265:G617–G625.

66   El-Salhy M, Sandstrom O, Holmlund F: Age-induced changes in the enteric nervous system in the mouse. Mech Ageing Dev 1999;107:93–103.
67   Gomes OA, de Souza RR, Liberti EA: A preliminary investigation of the effects of aging on the nerve cell number in the myenteric ganglia of the human colon. Gerontology 1997;43:210–217.
68   Camilleri M, Lee JS, Viramontes B, et al: Insights into the pathophysiology and mechanisms of constipation, irritable bowel syndrome and diverticulosis in older people. J Am Geriatr Soc 2000; 48:1142–1150.
69   Koch TR, Carney JA, Go VL, et al: Inhibitory neuropeptides and intrinsic inhibitory innervation of descending human colon. Dig Dis Sci 1991;36:712–718.
70   Takeuchi T, Niioka S, Yamaji M, et al: Decrease in participation of nitric oxide in nonadrenergic, noncholinergic relaxation of rat intestine with age. Jpn J Pharmacol 1998;78:293–302.

Alberto Pilotto
Unità Operativa Geriatria
Casa Sollievo della Sofferenza, Istituto di Ricovero e Cura a Carattere Scientifico
71013 San Giovanni Rotondo (FG) (Italy)
Tel./Fax +39 0882 410271, E-Mail alberto.pilotto@libero.it

Kuchel GA, Hof PR (eds): Autonomic Nervous System in Old Age.
Interdiscipl Top Gerontol. Basel, Karger, 2004, vol 33, pp 78–93

·······················

Structure and Function of the Aged Bladder

Cara Tannenbaum[a], *Qing Zhu*[b], *Jeff Ritchie*[b], *George A. Kuchel*[b]

[a]Institut universitaire de Gériatrie de Montréal, Université de Montréal, Montréal,
Québec, Canada, [b]UConn Center on Aging, University of Connecticut Health Center,
Farmington, Conn., USA

The human bladder is responsible for two functions: the storage of urine and voiding. These two seemingly simple functions require a high degree of complex physiologic coordination involving the bladder, its innervation as well as other organs [1]. Normal aging, as well as the presence of many disease processes which are common in old age can interact and impact upon bladder function and its overall capacity to maintain normal continence in old age. Moreover, any discussion of bladder function in old age is further complicated by the marked heterogeneity of the elderly population, particularly as pertains to overall health and the presence of concomitant illnesses or disabilities.

Factors Affecting Continence in the Elderly

Overall, the maintenance of continence in older individuals depends not only on a seamless integration of the autonomic and somatic nervous systems in bladder performance, but it also depends on many other factors, systems, and processes that extend beyond the bladder [2, 3]. For example, in many older individuals changes in mobility or fluid balance can be as important determinants of continence as are specific categories of bladder dysfunction. With these considerations in mind, any assessment of incontinent older individuals, particularly if they are frail, must also include an assessment of many relevant systems and functions other than the bladder. In fact, the scope and focus of such an evaluation does in some ways resemble that of a full geriatric assessment. Factors which may impact upon the ability of an older individual to remain continent and which need to be evaluated include mobility, medications, fluid balance, cardiac performance, plus disorders involving both the central and the peripheral nervous systems. Neurologic diseases require a particular attention, especially with respect to the possibility of cognitive deficits, abnormal spinal cord function and diminished lower extremity performance.

Physiologic and Functional Changes in the Aged Human Bladder

The natural history of bladder physiology and function in men and women has been examined in a number of clinical studies, nearly all cross-sectional. Moreover, data from healthy and/or continent elderly patients are few, making it difficult to assess the extent to which measurable age-associated changes in bladder function are primary aging phenomena, or possible consequences of diseases in old age. Nevertheless, some consistent changes appear to occur in parallel with normal aging. Specifically, changes in bladder contractility, capacity and stability (uninhibited detrusor contractions) will be discussed, as well as changes in anatomical and urodynamic parameters, and nocturnal fluid excretion patterns.

Symptoms of lower urinary tract dysfunction increase with age in both men and women, with increased urinary urgency frequency and nocturia occurring almost equally in men and women [4]. Urinary incontinence has been reported in up to 20% of community-dwelling men over age 65, with a prevalence more than twice as high in older women [5, 6]. In long-term care institutions, urinary incontinence afflicts 50% or more of elderly residents [7].

The range of normal bladder capacity varies considerably in younger individuals and values quoted for men lie between 350 and 750 ml and for women between 250 and 550 ml [8]. Although bladder capacity has been reported to decrease slightly with age [9], over 64% of continent, relatively healthy, community-dwelling elderly men were found to preserve a bladder capacity of 300 ml or more [10]. Among continent, relatively healthy, community-dwelling women over age 60, 70% had a bladder capacity of 300 ml or more [10]. Among individuals with uninhibited detrusor contractions, the mean bladder capacities of males and females were 323 and 364 ml, respectively, whereas for those who did not have any uninhibited detrusor contractions, mean bladder capacities were 419 and 404 ml [10]. In this study of 169 women and 94 men, an uninhibited bladder was estimated to occur in 35% of the male subjects, but only in 7.9% of female subjects. There was a tendency for uninhibited contractions to be greater for incontinent than for continent subjects, 50 vs. 32% in men and 12 vs. 5% in women. The higher prevalence of uninhibited contractions in men must be interpreted in light of the fact that the prostate enlarges in most older men and can cause uninhibited contractions and/or urodynamic obstruction in up to half of affected individuals [8, 11].

Detrusor contractility in the absence of uninhibited contractions has been reported to decrease slightly with age [9]. However, it should be noted that accurate contractility assessments present difficulties, particularly in the elderly and in the setting of bladder outlet obstruction [9]. Multiple methods based upon or applied during the pressure-flow study have been proposed for the assessment of detrusor contractility, but voiding efficiency from pressure-flow nomograms must be interpreted concomitantly with urethral resistance, which itself is hard to measure, especially when confounded by prostatic enlargement in men. Urine flow alone appears to decrease with age: for a minimum void of 200 ml, a minimally accepted maximum urine flow rate for men should be 21 ml/s for men aged 14–45, 12 ml/s for those aged 46–65, and 9 ml/s for those aged 66–80 [8]. For women with normal urinary tract function, normal flow rates decrease from 18 ml/s in women aged 14–45 and 15 ml/s in those aged 46 to 65, to 10 ml/s in those aged 66–80 [8]. However, these stated criteria for uroflowmetry normalcy are based on clinical experience and have not been validated in large longitudinal studies.

The postvoid residual urine volume (PVR) is another potential indicator of detrusor contractility. Mild, moderate and severe detrusor impairment, in the absence of outflow obstruction, abnormal straining or detrusor dyssynergia, have been defined by PVR values of 51–100, 101–250, and >250 ml, respectively [12, 13]. In studies of continent, community-dwelling elderly subjects, 25–86% of men and 50–78% of women had normal PVR values of less than 50 ml, with the remainder having various degrees of detrusor impairment [10, 14]. Maximal urethral pressure and functional urethral length also decrease in women with age [8, 15]; findings in men are more controversial because of the high prevalence of prostatic enlargement.

Finally, many normal physiological changes of aging affect the systems involved in urine formation and lead to nocturia in the elderly [16]. Diminished renal concentrating capacity, diminished sodium-conserving ability, loss of the circadian rhythm of antidiuretic hormone secretion, decreased secretion of renin-angiotensin-aldosterone, and increased secretion of atrial natriuretic hormone, all increase water excretion and nighttime urine production in older people. The constellation of increased nocturnal urine production and consequent nocturia with its associated effects on sleep disruption has been termed the 'nocturnal polyuria syndrome' [17, 18]. In young healthy persons there is a circadian pattern to urine production in which the ratio of daytime to nighttime urine production is usually greater than 2:1 and about 25% or less of daily urine output occurs during sleep. In persons over age 60, there is a reduction in the ratio of day to night urine flow to the point that nighttime flow rates become equal to or exceed the daytime rates [18]. Despite the change in the circadian pattern of urine excretion, total urine production per 24 h is not affected. Nonetheless, the interaction of nocturnal polyuria with age-associated decreases in bladder functional capacity and the higher prevalence of detrusor instability can make the older person particularly vulnerable to developing nocturnal urinary incontinence.

Normal Neural Control of the Bladder

In both humans and animals, neurologic control of the lower urinary tract and micturition is achieved via multiple reflex loops and neurotransmitters [1]. The detrusor and the outlet receive different innervations. Sacral parasympathetic (pelvic) nerves (S2–S4) provide an excitatory (muscarinic cholinergic and purinergic) input to the bladder, as well as an inhibitory (nitrergic) input to the urethra. Thoracolumbar sympathetic pathways (T11–L2), which release norepinephrine, provide an excitatory input to the bladder neck and urethra, as well as facilitatory and inhibitory input to parasympathetic ganglia. Lumbosacral efferent pathways (S3–S4) in pudendal nerves provide nicotinic cholinergic excitatory input to striated muscle in the urethral sphincter.

The most important afferent activity for initiating micturition arises in the bladder and passes through pelvic nerves to the sacral spinal cord. These afferents consist of small, myelinated (Aδ) fibers that respond in a graded manner to increasing intravesical pressure, the trigger pressure in humans being approximately 5–15 mm Hg. Both efferent and afferent spinal projections to the bladder by sympathetic, parasympathetic and somatic fibers overlap to a great extent. Along with connecting spinal interneurones, their cell bodies receive modulating signals from higher centers in the spinal cord, medulla, midbrain, diencephalon and cerebral cortex.

Normal neural control of the human bladder, urethra and associated sphincters is phasic unlike that observed in other autonomic systems which are tonically controlled. Thus, activities of their neural circuits vary greatly between the voiding or the storage phase. These two phases – voiding and storage – are felt to represent two mutually exclusive physiologic states. While the nature of the control and switching between these two states is not fully understood, it is felt to involve complex interactions between peripheral ganglia, the spinal cord, the brainstem and higher brain centers [19, 20].

Typically, during the bladder storage phase there is a low level of activity by vesical afferent and sacral parasympathetic outflow fibers. At the same time, there is a high level of activity by sympathetic and somatic fibers projecting to the internal and external sphincters, respectively. As a result of these changes, bladder storage is facilitated through an inhibition of the detrusor and of vesical parasympathetic ganglia. Urine storage mechanisms mediated by these sympathetic and somatic inputs to the urethral outlet are dependent upon spinal

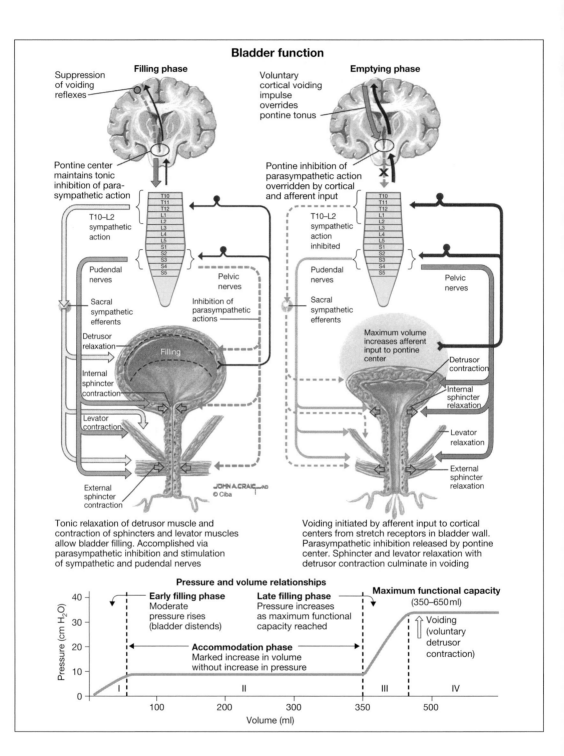

Bladder function

Filling phase

Suppression of voiding reflexes

Pontine center maintains tonic inhibition of parasympathetic action

T10–L2 sympathetic action

Pudendal nerves

Sacral sympathetic efferents

Detrusor relaxation

Internal sphincter contraction

Levator contraction

External sphincter contraction

Inhibition of parasympathetic actions

Pelvic nerves

Filling

JOHN A.CRAIG—AD
© Ciba

Tonic relaxation of detrusor muscle and contraction of sphincters and levator muscles allow bladder filling. Accomplished via parasympathetic inhibition and stimulation of sympathetic and pudendal nerves

Emptying phase

Voluntary cortical voiding impulse overrides pontine tonus

Pontine inhibition of parasympathetic action overridden by cortical and afferent input

T10–L2 sympathetic action inhibited

Pudendal nerves

Sacral sympathetic efferents

Maximum volume increases afferent input to pontine center

Pelvic nerves

Detrusor contraction

Internal sphincter relaxation

Levator relaxation

External sphincter relaxation

Voiding initiated by afferent input to cortical centers from stretch receptors in bladder wall. Parasympathetic inhibition released by pontine center. Sphincter and levator relaxation with detrusor contraction culminate in voiding

Pressure and volume relationships

Early filling phase
Moderate pressure rises (bladder distends)

Late filling phase
Pressure increases as maximum functional capacity reached

Maximum functional capacity
(350–650 ml)

Voiding (voluntary detrusor contraction)

Accommodation phase
Marked increase in volume without increase in pressure

I   II   III   IV

Pressure (cm H$_2$O): 0, 10, 20, 30, 40

Volume (ml): 100, 200, 300, 350, 500

reflex circuits, which are activated by sacral afferent nerve activity during bladder filling. During micturition, voiding reflexes involving activation of the parasympathetic input to the bladder and inhibition of the sympathetic and somatic inputs to the urethra, are mediated by a spinobulbospinal reflex pathway passing through a coordinating center in the rostral brain stem (the pontine micturition center). Modulation of the spinobulbospinal reflex circuit by higher centers in the cerebral cortex and diencephalons presumably underlies the voluntary control of voiding (fig. 1).

In summary, the bladder is predominantly innervated by parasympathetic and sensory nerves. Activation of parasympathetic pathways generally promotes bladder voiding by inducing detrusor contractions, as well as shortening and opening of the outlet (through contraction of longitudinal, rather than circular muscle), while activation of sympathetic pathways causes tonic constriction of the outlet and detrusor relaxation, both promoting urine storage and preventing leakage [20, 21]. Sensory pathways provide information relevant for micturition, and they may also convey nociceptive signals [22, 23].

The parasympathetic preganglionic neurons residing in the brain and the sacral spinal cord mediate parasympathetic outflow to the bladder. Cholinergic preganglionic neurons exit the spinal cord in the ventral spinal nerves to form the pelvic nerve, which then synapses on cholinergic postganglionic neurons in the major pelvic ganglia (MPG) residing in close proximity to the bladder [23]. Preganglionic fibers may also synapse on intramural ganglia within the bladder [24]. Bladder sympathetic innervation which is dominant in the outlet mostly arises from the sympathetic chain and is carried by the hypogastric and pelvic nerves to the detrusor and outlet [23]. Some also starts from inferior mesenteric ganglia which contribute exclusively to the detrusor, and from MPG projecting restrictly to the outlet [23]. The segmental locations of afferent nerves innervating the bladder detrusor and outlet are similar, with a slight predominance of the detrusor innervation by upper lumbar dorsal root ganglia (DRGs) and of outlet innervation by lumbar sacral DRGs. Overall, the majority of bladder afferent nerves localize their cell body at L6 DRG [23, 25]. Table 1 summarizes autonomic and sensory innervation of the bladder.

Autonomic nerve fibers and nerve terminals form a dense plexus among detrusor smooth muscle cells. Most of these nerves are excitatory cholinergic type [26]. EM studies of mammalian bladders have revealed the presence of a modest number of axons in all specimens. A variety of axon terminal profiles

Fig. 1. Bladder function. Reproduced from *Ciba Clinical Symposia* with kind permission from Novartis AG, Basel.

Table 1. Bladder innervation

Neurons	Type	Cell body	Detrusor	Outlet
Parasympathetic	efferent	MPG	++++	++
Sympathetic	efferent/afferent	SC, IMG, MPG	+(β)	+++(α)
Sensory	afferent	DRG (L6–S1)	+++	+++

were observed. Visible terminals included terminals which were bare and others which were either partially or completely ensheathed with Schwann cells [27, 28]. Cholinergic nerve terminals (with small clear synaptic vesicles) were the most frequently observed type of nerve terminal, while adrenergic axons (with small dense core synaptic vesicles) were rarely observed, particularly in the human detrusor [27, 29, 30].

Transmitters and Receptors

In mammals, acetylcholine has been proposed as the primary excitatory neurotransmitters for the activation of detrusor smooth muscle cells, through muscarinic acetylcholine receptor (mAChR) [31]. The density of mAChR on the surface of bladder smooth muscle cells and the responsiveness of these cells to acetylcholine stimulation are high in the dome and low in the base [29, 31], consistent with the innervation status mentioned previously [32]. The major subtypes of mAChR in the bladder have been shown to be M_2 and M_3 receptors based on their mRNA expression in porcine, rat and human bladders [33, 34].

It was proposed that the M_2 receptor exerts a modulatory action on β-adrenoceptor relaxant responses by inhibiting adenylyl cyclase activation [35]. Although M_3 receptor levels are lower than those of M_2, studies indicate that M_3 is the mediator of the direct contractile effect of acetylcholine in detrusor smooth muscle, acting through IP_3/Ca^{2+} signaling [35, 36]. Thus, during bladder voiding, M_3 receptor stimulation could produce direct contraction of the detrusor smooth muscle, whereas M_2 receptor may act indirectly by reversing sympathetically (β-adrenoceptor) induced relaxation of the smooth muscle. These two effects could synergize to produce a more efficient discharge of urine [37–39].

The majority of sympathetic activities in the bladder is mediated by α-adrenergic receptor which dominates in the outlet, and a small part by β-adrenergic receptor which mainly exists in the detrusor. Accordingly, there is evidence of 10-fold higher norepinephrine concentration and TH activity in the bladder outlet as compared to the detrusor [23, 25]. In addition to the above classical neurotransmitters, accumulating evidence points to the importance of an atropine insensitive, nonadrenergic, non-cholinergic neuronal component in bladder micturition mediated by ATP or purinergic analogs, acting mainly through P2X purinergic receptors consisting of subtypes [40, 41] including $P2X_{1-4}$ [40, 42]. The P2X receptors form ligand-gated cation channels through a novel trimeric subunit structure [43], and are responsible for depolarization of the cell membrane upon stimulation [27, 40, 43–50].

Effects of Aging on Bladder Innervation

Although a number of investigators have examined aging-associated changes in the mammalian bladder using established animal models, these findings have not been entirely consistent. For example, studies by Kolta et al. [51] showed an increased maximum contractile response in the whole bladder preparations elicited by cholinergic, but not adrenergic stimuli, which appeared to be a result of an increase in muscarinic receptor numbers. Whereas Hayes et al. [52] observed no age-related change in the density or affinity of muscarinic receptor by binding assay with the rat bladder. Dissection of the two regions (detrusor and outlet) revealed an age-related increase in the maximum contraction in response to α-adrenergic stimuli in the detrusor but not outlet [53]. Yet the increased responsiveness to cholinergic muscarinic was found in the outlet but not in the detrusor [54]. The discrepancies between the above-mentioned studies might be explained by differences in the rat strain, nature of tissue samples assayed, or/and the methods applied in different lab settings. These changes observed by Ordway et al. [53, 54] could not be explained by a change in the number or affinity of muscarinic receptors. It was proposed that post-receptor alterations such as that of coupling of activated receptor to contractile elements, or that of interactions of receptor with agonist or antagonist may account for the change of responsiveness [54]. The increased responsiveness of the bladder outlet to muscarinic responsiveness may indicate an increase in the tone of the smooth muscles in this region. Since the measured contraction was mainly by the longitudinal rather than circular outlet smooth muscle, and contraction of the former shortens the bladder outlet leading to opening of the outlet, geriatric urinary incontinence, might be related, among others, to the increased contractility in the outlet [54].

Comparison of the neurochemistry of the detrusor and outlet showed regional variations, but overall a number of cholinergic and sympathetic biochemical markers remain stable with advanced age [55]. In contrast, semiquantitative histochemical studies have revealed decreases in the sympathetic nerve bundles in both regions of the aged rat bladder (vs. 4 months old) with no significant changes in sensory fibers, suggesting that bladder sensory innervation is more resistant to the effects of advancing age [56].

Chun et al. [57] examined the effects of age on the in vivo bladder function in male rats, and revealed increased micturition volume and pressure at micturition, although no overt urological dysfunctions were observed in the aging rats. They then investigated the effects of aging on in vitro bladder function using a whole-bladder model [58]. It was demonstrated that bladder capacity did not change with aging, nor did the contractility of the bladder to autonomic agonists and nonautonomic drugs. The investigators therefore proposed that the age-related changes in micturition were due primarily to the alterations in neuronal innervation and central control rather than those in bladder contractility [58]. However, in vivo evidence presented by Hotta et al. [47] contradicted Chun et al. [58] in that they suggested changes in the mechanical properties and reduction in contractile capacity in the bladder with aging which coexist with innervation changes.

Ultrastructural Features of Normative Bladder Aging

In a recent series of urodynamic studies, normative bladder function has been defined by the absence of any detrusor hyperactivity, impaired detrusor contractility or bladder outlet obstruction in individuals 65 years old and older who have no evidence of any relevant neurologic disease [28]. Bladder biopsy studies have revealed that in these individuals the detrusor smooth muscle cells develop a 'dense-band pattern' which has been characterized by the presence of dense sarcolemmal bands in bladder muscle cells with markedly depleted caveolae (surface vesicles) [28]. It has been proposed that this depletion of caveolae may herald the 'dedifferentiation' of muscle cells from an active contractile phenotype to an inactive synthetic phenotype [9]. The spaces between aged bladder muscle cells are observed to be slightly widened (0.2–0.4 μm) with a limited increase in the content of collagen fibrils and rare, if any, elastic fibers. Apart from these changes, muscle fascicles generally preserve their normal arrangement and compact structure with cells retaining their cylindrical configuration, smooth contour, intermediate cell junctions and internal structure. Hypertrophic muscle cells are absent, and profiles of degenerating muscle cells and axons are absent or sparse.

Two variants of the normal aged detrusor have been described [13]. The first includes an incomplete dysjunction pattern characterized by abundant normal intermediate muscle-cell junctions with scattered protrusion junctions, not in chains. This incomplete pattern is distinct from the complete dysjunction pattern in which protrusion junctions and ultraclose abutments are much more abundant, often joining muscle cells in chains. The second variant is characterized by slightly increased muscle degeneration [13]. Intrinsic nerves in bladders from urodynamically normal older individuals appear normal [13, 28]. Although a few previous studies reported reduced density of intrinsic cholinergic nerves based on a method of nerve counting in aged detrusors, these studies have been questioned on methodological grounds [28, 59, 60].

All other structural abnormalities in aged bladders can be related to abnormal functional behavior on urodynamic evaluation. Three distinctive structural/functional correlates are worth mentioning because of their high prevalence in the elderly and their close association with urinary incontinence: the complete dysjunction pattern of the overactive detrusor with intact intrinsic nerve profiles, the full degeneration pattern of the muscle cells and intrinsic axons of the detrusor with impaired contractility, and the myohypertrophy pattern of the obstructed detrusor where the observed profiles of nerves and neuroeffector junctions appear normal [27, 28, 61]. The distinctive patterns of these various clinical and ultrastructural dysfunctions are additive when multiple abnormalities coexist.

In terms of the natural evolution of the aged detrusor, only one small follow-up study is available, but provides important insight into the progression of bladder function over time [13]. Among 23 detrusors in subjects aged 65–96 followed up over 1–5.5 years, 70% of the bladders remained unchanged clinically, urodynamically and structurally. The remaining 30% progressed both structurally and functionally in two different ways. The first, more common change involved the development of the complete dysjunction pattern in concert with urodynamic evidence of detrusor overactivity. In the second, a subject with a limited degeneration pattern progressed to a full degeneration pattern, coinciding with an increase in the impairment of detrusor contractility from mild to moderate. Although similar longitudinal studies in larger subject populations are needed to verify these findings, the results suggest that geriatric voiding function has some trends of natural evolution with time.

Changes in Bladder Morphology and Function in Aged Animals

There is a relative scarcity of published studies examining the effects of age alone on detrusor muscle. Most of these involve muscle strip studies, and some interesting results are discussed below. More commonly, animals are manipulated to reflect changes observed in human aging. These manipulations include ovariectomy to cause estrogen deficiency mimicking menopause, surgical bladder outlet obstruction, and streptozotocin-induced diabetes.

Generally it is found that with ageing, rat bladders increase in mass. Italiano et al. [48] found a 50% increase in bladder size from 6- to 27-month-old male Fischer 344 rats, while the rat body mass decreased by 13%. Lluel et al. [49] found an increase in the thickness of the muscularis layer from 10- to 30-month-old female Wistar rats, and they found that the amount of collagen detected by histological stains decreased. In contrast, in male and female Fischer 344 rats of 6 and 24 months, Longhurst et al. [50] using chemical assays found that both protein and collagen content increased with age. Also, these properties vary among different animals, even within the same species.

Using Muscle Strip and in vivo Contractility Studies

The effects of aging on the contractile properties and responsiveness of the bladder appear to vary between experimental models and also between different regions of the same bladder.

In conscious Wistar Wag/Rij rats, Lluel et al. [49] found that while aged animals had more spontaneous contractions during the bladder-filling phase, and significantly higher pressure and duration of micturition, there was no significant difference in bladder capacity, bladder compliance, micturition volume or residual volume. In these animals, the contractile responses of the bladder body muscle strips to KCl, carbachol, arecoline and α,β-methyl ATP remained similar, while the maximal response to noradrenaline doubled. Relaxation of precontracted muscle by isoprenaline did not change. The detrusor instability and increased response to α-adrenergic agonists mimic changes seen in aged human bladders, but other changes, such as decreased compliance, are not seen in this breed.

In contrast to the absence of changes in compliance with aging in Wistar rats, Pagala et al. [62] suggested that there are changes in the compliance of the circular running muscle fibers of male Fischer 344 rats. This conclusion was drawn from observations that responsiveness to electrical field stimulation increased while the response to bethanechol decreased. Different age-dependent changes were observed in different regions of the bladder. Consistent with previous studies, they found decrease responsiveness to bethanechol but not high potassium and electrical field stimulation, indicating a reduction in the number of muscarinic receptors, while they found a decreased response to all of these stimuli in the trigone.

Also in contrast to the results of Lluel et al. [49] in Wistar rats, Saito et al. [63, 64] found that anesthetized 24-month-old male Sprague-Dawley rats voided with a significantly lower pressure than their 6-month-old counterparts. The blood flow in the bladder was reduced in older animals, and both young and old animals exhibited reduced blood flow to the bladder upon filling.

Muscle strip studies by Lin et al. [65] document a more rapid fatigue in response to electrical field stimulation in detrusor from old rats. In a follow-up study, they relate this to a reduction in mitochondrial enzyme activity and a reduced ability to generate energy in the form of ATP and phosphocreatine. A review by Nevel-McGarvey et al. [66] discusses mitochondria and bladder dysfunction.

Role of Hormones in Aging- and Menopause-Associated Changes

Studies with middle-aged rats by Zhu et al. [67] demonstrated that bilateral ovariectomy causing prolonged estrogen deficiency in aged rats mimics some of the ultrastructural features observed by Elbadawi et al. [28] in 'idiopathic' impaired contractility in many older individuals. The changes observed in these ovariectomized rats included degeneration involving many, but not all, axons in the bladder, decreased smooth muscle content, and a reduction in tension generated by muscle strips in response to carbachol in ovariectomized animals compared to age-matched sham operated controls. A study by Diep et al. [68] highlights the importance of the age at which ovariectomy and E_2 replacement are performed, showing that 2-month-old animals respond differently to ovariectomy and E_2 than mature 10-month-old rats do. In studies where understanding conditions affecting the elderly is a primary goal, it is important that manipulations be performed after maturity, to avoid potential confounding developmental effects.

Use of the Acute Bladder Obstruction Animal Model of Bladder Plasticity

Surgically restricting the diameter of the bladder outlet and urethra leads to dramatic changes that depend on the degree of obstruction, and mimic functional and morphological changes seen in conditions of human bladder outlet obstruction, such as benign prostatic hypertrophy. This model has been extensively studied, and changes observed include myohypertrophy, urodynamically demonstrated detrusor instability. Kohan et al. [69] found changes in bladder function with both outlet obstruction and with age, as well as changes in response to outlet obstruction with age in obstructed and age-matched control 6-, 12-, 18- and 24-month-old female Fischer 344 rats. They found significant decreases in compliance with age, while bladder outlet obstruction caused severe instability, increased compliance and increased capacity. In response to outlet obstruction, young animals produced a compensatory increase in voiding pressure, while older animals did not.

A study by Yu et al. [70] investigated voiding against high outlet resistance by young (6 months) and old (3 years) rabbit bladders in vitro found that maximum power remained constant with varied outlet resistance for a given age. The maximum power was decreased in older animals, and could not be maintained long enough to fully void against increased resistance. As a result of these observations, the authors suggested that determining maximum bladder power independently of resistance might be clinically useful, and that taking voided volume into account, bladder work could also be a useful concept.

The different changes in bladder compliance that occur in different rat breeds with aging, combined with the knowledge that changes occur in compliance with variables such as high outlet resistance, illustrate the complexity of studying normal aging. Even in the relatively uniform lives of lab animals, there are many uncontrolled variables, including potential differences in diet, animal care, confounding pathology and strain-specific genetic backgrounds that can make comparisons between results obtained in different studies difficult.

Despite the apparent simplicity of normal bladder function, the bladder requires complex innervation regulating storage and micturition, and numerous factors affect continence status in the elderly. Differences in capacity, contractility and stability have been studied in the elderly, but variability is high. Ultrastructural studies of the aging human bladder have however permitted the description of superimposable patterns – the dense band, complete dysjunction and degenerative patterns – correlating respectively with normative aging, detrusor overactivity and impaired contractility. The results of experiments examining the effects of age on innervation and physiology of the bladder in animal models appear to be dependent on the genetic background of the animals, and on the regions of the bladder studied. It is clearly important that all animal models used in aging studies be well characterized, and carefully selected to most closely resemble the human phenomenon of interest.

References

1   De Groat WC, Yoshimura N: Pharmacology of the lower urinary tract. Annu Rev Pharmacol Toxicol 2001;41:691.
2   Resnick NM: Urinary incontinence. Lancet 1995;346:94.
3   Tannenbaum C, Perrin L, DuBeau CE, Kuchel GA: Diagnosis and management of urinary incontinence in the older patient. Arch Phys Med Rehabil 2001;82:134.
4   Homma Y, Imajo C, Takahashi S, Kawabe K, Aso Y: Urinary symptoms and urodynamics in a normal elderly population. Scand J Urol Nephrol Suppl 1994;157:27.
5   Roberts RO, Jacobsen SJ, Rhodes T, Reilly WT, Girman CJ, Talley NJ, et al: Urinary incontinence in a community-based cohort: Prevalence and healthcare-seeking. J Am Geriatr Soc 1998;46:467.
6   Thom D: Variation in estimates of urinary incontinence prevalence in the community: Effects of differences in definition, population characteristics, and study type. J Am Geriatr Soc 1998; 46:473.

7   Fantl JA, Newman DK, Colling J: Urinary incontinence in adults: Acute and chronic management. Clinical Practice Guideline No 2. AHCPR Publication No 96–0682. Rockville, MD, US. Department of Health and Human Services. Public Health Service. Agency for Health Care Policy and Research, 1996.

8   Abrams P, Feneley R, Torrens M: Urodynamics. New York, Springer, 1983.

9   Elbadawi A, Diokno AC, Millard RJ: The aging bladder: Morphology and urodynamics. World J Urol 1998;16(suppl 1):S10.

10   Diokno AC, Brown MB, Brock BM, Herzog AR, Normolle DP: Clinical and cystometric characteristics of continent and incontinent noninstitutionalized elderly. J Urol 1988;140:567.

11   Isaacs JT, Coffey DS: Etiology and disease process of benign prostatic hyperplasia. Prostate Suppl 1989;2:33.

12   Elbadawi A, Yalla SV, Resnick NM: Structural basis of geriatric voiding dysfunction. I. Methods of a prospective ultrastructural/urodynamic study and an overview of the findings. J Urol 1993; 150:1650.

13   Elbadawi A, Hailemariam S, Yalla SV, Resnick NM: Structural basis of geriatric voiding dysfunction. VII. Prospective ultrastructural/urodynamic evaluation of its natural evolution. J Urol 1997; 157:1814.

14   Bonde HV, Sejr T, Erdmann L, Meyhoff HH, Lendorf A, Rosenkilde P, et al: Residual urine in 75-year-old men and women. A normative population study. Scand J Urol Nephrol 1996; 30:89.

15   Rud T: Urethral pressure profile in continent women from childhood to old age. Acta Obstet Gynecol Scand 1980;59:331.

16   Miller M: Nocturnal polyuria in older people: Pathophysiology and clinical implications. J Am Geriatr Soc 2000;48:1321.

17   Asplund R: The nocturnal polyuria syndrome (NPS). Gen Pharmacol 1995;26:1203.

18   Kirkland JL, Lye M, Levy DW, Banerjee AK: Patterns of urine flow and electrolyte excretion in healthy elderly people. Br Med J (Clin Res Ed) 1983;287:1665.

19   De Groat WC, Booth AM: Synaptic transmission in pelvic ganglia; in Maggi CA (ed): The Autonomic Nervous System, vol 3: Nervous Control of the Urogenital System. London, Harwood Academic Publishers, 1993, p 291.

20   De Groat WC: Neuroanatomy and neurophysiology: Innervation of the lower urinary tract; in Raz S (ed): Female Urology. Philadelphia, Saunders, 1995, p 28.

21   Levin RM, Wein AJ: Distribution and function of adrenergic receptors in the urinary bladder. Mol Pharmacol 1979;16:441.

22   de Groat WC: Nervous control of the urinary bladder of the cat. Brain Res 1975;87:201.

23   Vera PL, Nadelhaft I: Afferent and sympathetic innervation of the dome and the base of the urinary bladder of the female rat. Brain Res Bull 1992;29:651.

24   Chai TC, Steers WD: Neurophysiology of micturition and continence. Urol Clin North Am 1996; 23:221.

25   Vera PL, Nadelhaft I: Conduction velocity distribution of afferent fibers innervating the rat urinary bladder. Brain Res 1990;520:83.

26   Dixon JS, Gosling JA: Ultrastructure of smooth muscle cells in the urinary system; in Motta PM (ed): Ultrastructure of Smooth Muscle. Boston, Kluwer, 1990, p 153.

27   Elbadawi A, Yalla SV, Resnick NM: Structural basis of geriatric voiding dysfunction. IV. Bladder outlet obstruction. J Urol 1993;150:1681.

28   Elbadawi A, Yalla SV, Resnick NM: Structural basis of geriatric voiding dysfunction. II. Aging detrusor: Normal versus impaired contractility. J Urol 1993;150:1657.

29   McConnell J, Benson GS, Wood JG: Autonomic innervation of the urogenital system: Adrenergic and cholinergic elements. Brain Res Bull 1982;9:679.

30   Resnick NM, Yalla SV: Management of urinary incontinence in the elderly. N Engl J Med 1985; 313:800.

31   Chai TC, Steers WD: Neurophysiology of micturition and continence. Urol Clin North Am 1996; 23:221.

32   Levin RM, Shofer FS, Wein AJ: Estrogen-induced alterations in the autonomic responses of the rabbit urinary bladder. J Pharmacol Exp Ther 1980;215:614.

33   Maeda A, Kubo T, Mishina M, Numa S: Tissue distribution of mRNAs encoding muscarinic acetylcholine receptor subtypes. FEBS Lett 1988;239:339.

34   Wall SJ, Yasuda RP, Li M, Wolfe BB: Development of an antiserum against M_3 muscarinic receptors: Distribution of M_3 receptors in rat tissues and clonal cell lines. Mol Pharmacol 1991;40:783.

35   Longhurst PA, Leggett RE, Briscoe JA: Characterization of the functional muscarinic receptors in the rat urinary bladder. Br J Pharmacol 1995;116:2279.

36   Berridge MJ, Dupont G: Spatial and temporal signalling by calcium. Curr Opin Cell Biol 1994; 6:267.

37   Wang P, Luthin GR, Ruggieri MR: Muscarinic acetylcholine receptor subtypes mediating urinary bladder contractility and coupling to GTP binding proteins. J Pharmacol Exp Ther 1995;273:959.

38   Hegde SS, Choppin A, Bonhaus D, Briaud S, Loeb M, Moy TM, et al: Functional role of M_2 and M_3 muscarinic receptors in the urinary bladder of rats in vitro and in vivo. Br J Pharmacol 1997;120:1409.

39   Mimata H, Nomura Y, Emoto A, Latifpour J, Wheeler M, Weiss RM: Muscarinic receptor subtypes and receptor-coupled phosphatidylinositol hydrolysis in rat bladder smooth muscle. Int J Urol 1997;4:591.

40   Theobald RJ Jr: Purinergic and cholinergic components of bladder contractility and flow. Life Sci 1995;56:445.

41   Tong YC, Hung YC, Shinozuka K, Kunitomo M, Cheng JT: Evidence of adenosine 5'-triphosphate release from nerve and P2x-purinoceptor mediated contraction during electrical stimulation of rat urinary bladder smooth muscle. J Urol 1997;58:1973.

42   Dutton JL, Hansen MA, Balcar VJ, Barden JA, Bennett MR: Development of P2X receptor clusters on smooth muscle cells in relation to nerve varicosities in the rat urinary bladder. J Neurocytol 1999;28:4.

43   Nicke A, Baumert HG, Rettinger J, Eichele A, Lambrecht G, Mutschler E, et al: P2X1 and P2X3 receptors form stable trimers: A novel structural motif of ligand-gated ion channels. EMBO J 1998;17:3016.

44   North RA, Barnard EA: Nucleotide receptors. Curr Opin Neurobiol 1997;7:346.

45   Hoyle CH, Burnstock G: Atropine-resistant excitatory junction potentials in rabbit bladder are blocked by alpha,beta-methylene ATP. Eur J Pharmacol 1985;114:239.

46   Chancellor MB, Kaplan SA, Blaivas JG: The cholinergic and purinergic components of detrusor contractility in a whole rabbit bladder model. J Urol 1992;148:906.

47   Hotta H, Morrison JF, Sato A, Uchida S: The effects of aging on the rat bladder and its innervation. Jpn J Physiol 1995;45:823.

48   Italiano G, Calabro A, Artibani W, Cisternino A, Oliva G, Pagano F: Bladder function in the aged rat: A functional and morphological study. Eur Urol 1995;27:232.

49   Lluel P, Palea S, Barras M, Grandadam F, Heudes D, Bruneval P, et al: Functional and morphological modifications of the urinary bladder in aging female rats. Am J Physiol Regul Integr Comp Physiol 2000;278:R964.

50   Longhurst PA, Eika B, Leggett RE, Levin RM: Comparison of urinary bladder function in 6 and 24 month male and female rats. J Urol 1992;148:1615.

51   Kolta MG, Wallace LJ, Gerald MC: Age-related changes in sensitivity of rat urinary bladder to autonomic agents. Mech Ageing Dev 1984;27:183.

52   Hayes EE, McConnell JA, Benson GS: The effect of aging on cholinergic receptor binding in the rat urinary bladder. Neurourol Urodyn 1983;2:311.

53   Ordway GA, Kolta MG, Gerald MC, Wallace LJ: Age-related change in alpha-adrenergic responsiveness of the urinary bladder of the rat is regionally specific. Neuropharmacology 1986;25:1335.

54   Ordway GA, Esbenshade TA, Kolta MG, Gerald MC, Wallace LJ: Effect of age on cholinergic muscarinic responsiveness and receptors in the rat urinary bladder. J Urol 1986;136:492.

55   Johnson JM, Skau KA, Gerald MC, Wallace LJ: Regional noradrenergic and cholinergic neurochemistry in the rat urinary bladder: Effects of age. J Urol 1988;139:611.

56   Warburton AL, Santer RM: Sympathetic and sensory innervation of the urinary tract in young adult and aged rats: A semi-quantitative histochemical and immunohistochemical study. Histochem J 1994;26:127.

57   Chun AL, Wallace LJ, Gerald MC, Levin RM, Wein AJ: Effect of age on in vivo urinary bladder function in the rat. J Urol 1988;139:625.
58   Chun AL, Wallace LJ, Gerald MC, Wein AJ, Levin RM: Effects of age on urinary bladder function in the male rat. J Urol 1989;141:170.
59   Canon E, Timmermans LG, Reznik M, Timmermans LM: Ultrastructural modifications of the bladder wall in senescence. Acta Urol Belg 1990;58:29.
60   Martin D, Vaira S, Timmermans LMJ: Changes in bladder intrinsic innervation during senescence. CR Soc Biol 1985;179:501.
61   Elbadawi A, Yalla SV, Resnick NM: Structural basis of geriatric voiding dysfunction. III. Detrusor overactivity. J Urol 1993;150:1668.
62   Pagala MK, Tetsoti L, Nagpal D, Wise GJ: Aging effects on contractility of longitudinal and circular detrusor and trigone of rat bladder. J Urol 2001;166:721.
63   Saito M, Gotoh M, Kato K, Kondo A: Influence of aging on the rat urinary bladder function. Urol Int 1991;47(suppl 1):39.
64   Saito M, Ohmura M, Kondo A: Effect of ageing on blood flow to the bladder and bladder function. Urol Int 1999;62:93.
65   Lin AT, Yang CH, Chang LS: Impact of aging on rat urinary bladder fatigue. J Urol 1997; 157:1990.
66   Nevel-McGarvey CA, Levin RM, Haugaard N, Wu X, Hudson AP: Mitochondrial involvement in bladder function and dysfunction. Mol Cell Biochem 1999;194:1.
67   Zhu Q, Ritchie J, Marouf N, Dion SB, Resnick NM, Elbadawi A, et al: Role of ovarian hormones in the pathogenesis of impaired detrusor contractility: Evidence from ovariectomized rodents. J Urol 2001;166:1136.
68   Diep N, Constantinou CE: Age dependent response to exogenous estrogen on micturition, contractility and cholinergic receptors of the rat bladder. Life Sci 1999;64:PL279–PL289.
69   Kohan AD, Danziger M, Vaughan ED Jr, Felsen D: Effect of aging on bladder function and the response to outlet obstruction in female rats. Urol Res 2000;28:33.
70   Yu HJ, Levin RM, Longhurst PA, Damaser MS: Effect of age and outlet resistance on rabbit urinary bladder emptying. J Urol 1997;158:924.

George A. Kuchel, MD
Director, UConn Center on Aging
University of Connecticut Health Center
MC-5215, 263 Farmington Ave., Farmington, CT 06030–5215 (USA)
Tel. +1 860 679 3956, Fax +1 860 679 1307, E-Mail kuchel@nso1.uchc.edu

Kuchel GA, Hof PR (eds): Autonomic Nervous System in Old Age.
Interdiscipl Top Gerontol. Basel, Karger, 2004, vol 33, pp 94–106

....

Impact of Aging on Reproduction and Sexual Function

Evette Beshay, Khaleeq-ur-Rehman, Serge Carrier

McGill University Health Center, Royal Victoria Hospital, McGill University,
Montreal, Quebec, Canada

Aging and Reproduction

Median human survival has greatly increased during recent decades. As a consequence of the resulting demographic changes, issues relevant to reproductive aging have assumed a major importance in today's society. The issue of fertility in aging has received increase attention due to several factors. In industrialized developed countries, family planning often begins after the establishment of both parents' careers, resulting in increasingly higher parental ages. This attitude is often triggered by socioeconomic factors. One of the other factors involved has been the advancement in assisted reproduction techniques, particularly intracytoplasmic sperm injection (ICSI), which has led to significant improvement in fertilization and pregnancy rates, offering the possibility of parenthood to couples who in the past would have not been able to conceive.

Effect of Aging on Female Fertility

It is well recognized that the reproductive potential of women declines with age. Age-related change in the ovary accounts for most of the loss in reproductive function. There is a marked decline in the number and quality of oocytes with age and the ovary becomes unable to sustain its normal function in the neuroendocrine axis [1]. Aging also directly affects both uterine structure (loss of endometrium), as well as function (loss of its ability to support implantation).

Declines in uterine function associated with aging are mediated by age-related changes in uterine vasculature, as well as diminished hormonal support for the endometrium [2, 3].

The decline of women's fertility begins at 30 years of age, with few women remaining fertile by 45 [4]. This phenomenon has been observed for both natural conception and assisted reproduction. A pioneering study of natural conception investigated a group of Hutterite women who belong to a Protestant sect that condemns the practice of contraception. The mean age of last confinement was 41 and the interval between confinements increased with advancing maternal age [5]. The same trend has been noted in women undergoing assisted reproductive technologies. In women older than 35 years, the success rate after assisted reproductive technology starts to decline, and by the age of 40 a marked decline in success rates is noted [6–8]. Several studies of artificial insemination showed that the cumulative pregnancy rate decreases significantly as the age of the women increases [9–13]. The pregnancy rate achieved by in vitro fertilization (IVF) and gamete intrafallopian transfer has also been shown to decrease in older women [13–17].

Effect of Aging on Male Fertility

Unlike female fertility, which ends at the entrance into menopause, men generally do not experience an unavoidable and clear-cut cessation of reproductive capacity. Unfortunately, there are no longitudinal studies available to demonstrate the effect of aging in male fertility.

However, morphological alterations of the testis with aging have been described. It has been shown that the number of Leydig cells which are responsible for testosterone production are reduced and that thickening and hernia-like protrusion of the basal membrane of the seminiferous tubules occur [18–20]. The presence of areas with disturbances of spermatogenesis has also been reported [21]. It has been proposed that a reduction in testicular perfusion, together with arteriosclerotic lesions of the testicular arterioles, contributes to diminished spermatogenesis in older men. However, a study examining parenchymal testicular weight observed no difference between men aged 21–50 years and those 51–80 years old [20]. It was assumed that with increasing age, new layers of connective tissue are deposited, leading to thickening of the tunica albuginea. With aging, testicular volume, blood flow, daily production of spermatozoa and the number of Leydig cells are reduced [22]. Also, it has been reported in other species, like the horse, that the testis develops interstitial fibrosis and atrophic changes in seminiferous tubules during aging [23].

The effect of paternal age on fertilization and pregnancy rates has received increasing attention following the development of improvements in assisted reproduction techniques by using ICSI. This technique enables selective fertilization of a single oocyte with a single vital sperm via a microinjection pipette. The pregnancy rate after intercourse, intrauterine insemination, in vitro fertilization, and ICSI were investigated in three groups: group 1 – young men and women; group 2 – young men and older women and group 3 – older men and older women [24]. The pregnancy rate was significantly higher in group 1, but no significant difference was seen between groups 2 and 3. Men remain fertile with aging and the age of the female partner seemed to be the most important in predicting the reproductive chance of a couple. The pregnancy outcome of ICSI was related to maternal but not paternal age [25].

Semen Parameters in Elderly Men

On the basis of cross-sectional studies, alterations of semen parameters such as motility and sperm count have been described. However, semen analysis demonstrates a lot of variation in sperm quality when obtaining a sample from the same individual on different occasions. This high intraindividual variability in semen quality makes research into the effects of aging on semen parameters difficult. As a result, any crosssectional studies based on a single semen parameter should be interpreted with caution [26]. A previous study has reported that there is no significant difference in semen volume, sperm count, or the total number of spermatozoa in over 800 fertile men studied between the ages of 21 and 50 [27]. Elderly men were not included in this study. Other studies reported significant increases in sperm density in older men (60- to 88-year-old) [28]. However, several studies that included different age groups showed no significant changes in sperm concentration [27, 29]. Reduction in sperm motility with aging has also been reported in several studies [27, 28, 30]. In contrast, Haidle et al. [31] reported a reduction in sperm concentration in older fathers (mean age 50.3 years) as compared to younger fathers (mean age 32.2 years), with no apparent differences in acrosomal reaction or chromatin condensation of human spermatozoa.

Paternal Age and Birth Defect

The genetic quality of sperm produced by older men may be reduced for several reasons. Among the factors contributing to declines in genetic quality of sperm from older men are age-related increases in germ cell mutations, impaired DNA repair mechanisms, alterations in apoptotic processes, as well as increased DNA transcription error rate with paternal aging. An increased risk of genetic disorders and autosomal dominant diseases known to occur in offsprings of older men is a direct consequence of altered genetic sperm quality [32–34]. Older fathers have a greater risk of conceiving children with birth defects. Children of older men are at a particularly great risk of developing ventricular septal defects, atrial septal defects, chondrodystrophy, in situs inversus, polycystic kidneys, Marfan's syndrome, as well as polyposis coli [32–34]. In view of these findings, the American Fertility Society recommended that semen donors for intrauterine insemination be 50 years of age or younger in order to minimize the risk of chromosomal abnormalities and birth defects [35].

Endocrinology of Aging

Andropause
A progressive decline in androgen production has been described with aging, and has been termed the andropause. In many ways, the term andropause is biologically incorrect and clinically inappropriate, yet it does convey adequately the concept of the emotional and physical changes related to aging. Hormonal changes associated with the andropause may contribute to the following key aging changes: (1) decreased sexual desire and erectile quality particularly during nocturnal erection; (2) changes in mood, decreased intellectual function, fatigue, depression and anger; (3) decreased lean body mass with diminished muscle volume and strength; (4) decreased body hair and skin alterations, and (5) decreased bone mineral density plus increased visceral fat (table 1) [36].

Changes in the activity of the hypothalamo-pituitary-gonadal axis in aging men occur and are associated with a gradual decline in both total and free serum testosterone levels. Aging is characterized by a decrease in testicular Leydig cell number and their secretory capacity, as well as an age-related decrease in episodic and stimulated gonadotropin secretion [37]. It has been proposed that, as a general rule of thumb, mean serum testosterone decreases by approximately 1% per year after the age of 50. However, large interindividual variations exist. True biochemical hypogonadism is detected in only 7% of men younger than 60 years, with rates increasing to 20% in those older than 60 [37]. An increase in sex hormone-binding globulin occurs with advancing age and translates into a further decrease in testosterone bioavailable (free and albumin bond fraction) [37].

Table 1. Characteristics of andropause

Decreases in sexual desire
Decreases in erectile function
Changes in mood
Decreases in intellectual capacity/activity
Decrease in lean body mass
Decreases in muscle volume
Decreases in body hair
Alterations of the skin
Decreases in bone mineral density
Increases in visceral fat

Menopause

In contrast to men, women experience dramatic and rapid changes in their hormonal status around the age of 50 years old (menopause). At that time, ovarian production of estrogen ceases. Many, but not all, postmenopausal women experience a marked reduction in serum estradiol (E_2) levels. For many years, the prevailing view was that menopause resulted from the exhaustion of the ovarian follicles. An alternative perspective is that age-related changes in the central nervous system and the hypothalamo-pituitary axis initiate the transition to menopause [38]. Menopause and andropause have a tremendous impact on sexual function. They both have a negative effect on libido or sexual desire. The andropause can, furthermore, have a negative impact on men's erectile function whereas, while menopause can hamper lubrication or the arousal phase in women.

Aging and Sexual Function in Men

Over the past decade, a better understanding of the pathophysiology of erectile dysfunction has led to the discovery of new therapy. Sildenafil (Viagra®), the first oral phosphodiesterase type 5 inhibitor, has revolutionized and eased the treatment of erectile dysfunction. Studies have shown that although erectile dysfunction is not caused by aging, its prevalence definitively increases with age. According to the Massachusetts Male Aging Study, the annual incidence rate of erectile dysfunction increases with every decade of life, with an annual incidence rate of 12.4 per 1,000 man-years for men between the age of 40–49, 29.8 between 50–59 and 46.4 between the age of 60–69 [39]. At 70 years of age, close to 2 out of 3 men have some degree of erectile dysfunction. With the population aging and a growing emphasis being placed on quality of life,

---

the demand for impotence evaluation and treatment will continue to increase in the future. Although, aging is by itself not responsible for erectile dysfunction, men are going through physiological changes that may alter the sexual response.

Sexual Desire

Sex continues to be important in elderly men. More than 83% of 50- to 80-year-old Swedish men consider sex to be important for them. Among the same group, 46% of men reported to have orgasm at least once a month [40]. In older men, however, a decrease in libido can be induced by a decrease in testosterone level as discussed above [41]. Although libido and sexual desire are linked to androgen levels, other factors such as chronic illnesses may also impact [42–44]. Unfavorable social circumstances such as living in nursing home, diseases like diabetes, medications such as antidepressant and anti-hypertensive drugs or the use of alcohol, can all contribute to the diminution of sexual desire and function [45].

Sexual and Orgasmic Function

In aged rats, changes in sexual function can be demonstrated. The first change is a decrease in erectile reflexes followed by a decrease in ejaculatory threshold and an abnormal delay in initiating and reinitiating copulation after ejaculation and a decreased number of males reaching ejaculation. Finally, there is a failure to initiate the copulatory process [46]. The kinetics of erection and detumescence are also lower in aging rats [47]. These changes also occur in older men. With aging, the orgasms become less intense, brief and less frequent [48]. The sexual reaction and intensity of ejaculation are slowed down and ejaculation is less forceful [49]. A reduction of the semen volume is noticed and is more apparent when comparing 30-year-old men to 50-year-olds [48, 50]. The refractory period (the period following an orgasm when a man cannot obtain a second erection) also increases with age. It can be as much as 48 h in an 80-year-old man (table 2). The use of medications such as antidepressants may further alter this impairment of function in elderly males. Some of them even develop anorgasmia [51].

Aging produces degenerative and structural alterations of the elastic fibers in the corporal tissue as well as in the tunica albuginea [47]. There is a reduced concentration of elastic fibers in the tunica albuginea that may lead to the impairment of the veno-occlusive mechanism [52, 53]. Atherosclerotic changes develop in the penis with age leading to a decrease in corporal oxygen tension. Chronic ischemia

Table 2. Changes in sexual function with age

Decreases in frequency and intensity of orgasm
Decreases in intensity and force of ejaculation
Decreases in semen volume
Increases in refractory period
Decreases of penile rigidity in erection
Decreases in penile sensation
  Needs more sexual stimulation
    To get an erection
    To maintain an erection

results in fibrosis of the corporal structure. This injury also leads to disturbance in both neurological and endothelial elements. The nitric oxide (NO)/cGMP pathway is also affected by these changes. We have shown a decrease in NO synthase (NOS)-containing nerve fibers in rat penis with age [54]. These changes explain the evolution of the sexual function associated with aging. Impairment in penile collagen turnover develops with aging. This has been observed in cadaver as well as living tissue. There is a 6-fold increase in the levels of pentosidine, an advanced glycation end product in the tunica albuginea and a 4-fold increase in corpora from puberty to 100 years of age. Transforming growth factor-β1 (TGFβ1) gene expression is significantly increased in aging rat penile tissue [55]. These changes could explain the decrease in the elasticity of tunica albuginea occurring with age and the decrease in overall rigidity of the penis. In aging, as in diabetes, nonenzymatic glycation of proteins forms proteins and DNA adducts and cross-links which, by scavenging NO, may contribute to sexual dysfunction [56].

A downregulation of NO activity is also seen in castrated rats, which is upregulated after immediate or delayed testosterone replacement [57]. Even after 8 weeks' delay in testosterone replacement a similar improvement in erectile function has been observed in castrated rats [58]. In man, testosterone levels gradually decrease with age. The fall in testosterone could decrease the overall NO activity with age and explain in part the decrease in erectile ability. All these changes lead to a decrease in the overall rigidity of the erect penis in aging (table 2). The reduced rigidity seen in the aging penis should not, however, interfere with penetration in the elderly.

Aging and Penile Sensations

The penile sensory afferent pathway is through the pudendal nerve. Penile sensations diminish with aging. This sensory deficit correlates with erectile dysfunction [59, 60]. Pudendal neuropathy and decreased pudendal nerve conduction have been associated with aging [61, 62]. Human pudendal nerve terminal latency increases with age, with individual values ranging from 1.8 to 5.6 ms in men between the ages of 21 and 75 [63]. In rats, we have demonstrated that the delay before the intracavernosal pressure rises after cavernous nerve electrostimulation increased with age from 2.3 ± 0.24 s in young adults to 6.77 ± 0.98 s in older rats [54].

Decreases in vibrotactile sensitivity have also been shown in older rats. Single penile mechanoreceptor efferent fibers exhibit an inability to transmit high frequency vibratory stimuli as compared to the controls. A reduction in single fiber and sensory nerve conduction velocity was also noted [64]. In aging, the terminal axons of the sympathetic autonomic ganglion are markedly swollen and argyrophilic and a large number of microfilaments are observed in the ganglia [65]. These changes reflect the needs of more sexual stimulation for older men to get and maintain an erection comparable to younger men (table 2).

Aging and Central Nervous System

Aging has been associated with andropause, menopause, adrenopause and somatopause (decrease in the adrenal and the thyroid function, respectively). As a result of these widespread hormonal changes, it has been hypothesized that a central pacemaker, possibly located in the hypothalamus or higher brain areas, may set the clock for age-related changes in various components of the endocrine axis. A single deficit in this pacemaker occurring with aging could be responsible for these different clinical entities [38]. Oxytocinergic neurons of the paraventricular nucleus of the hypothalamus have a modulating effect on the male sexual response. Destruction of these neurons leads to decreased seminal emission during ejaculation in rats [66]. Oxytocin stimulates the behavior of aging male rats. It shortens the latencies for mount, intromission, ejaculation and postejaculation interval. A decrease in oxytocin has been postulated to explain the decrease in their ejaculatory function with age [67].

In aging rats with sexual dysfunction, grafting of fetal hypothalamic tissue into the third ventricle leads to a restoration of sexual behavior. The preoptic area appears to be involved in the age-related decrease in copulatory activity and sexual motivation [68]. Stroke is a common cause of disability in the aging population [69]. Sexual dysfunction is common in men and women after a cerebrovascular injury [70]. The majority of men (50–65%) will have erectile dysfunction after a stroke. This is particularly true when the dominant hemisphere is injured [71–73]. Injury to the frontal and temporal lobe appear to induce more sexual problems than lesion to the parieto-occipital region of the brain. Hemianesthesia or hypoaesthesia decrease sexual ability due probably to the loss of erogenous zones.

Aging and Sexual Function in Women

With age, women go through more drastic hormonal changes than men do; Obviously menopause has a significant impact on sexual function. Common sexual complaints associated with aging and decrease in estrogen level include loss of desire, decreased frequency of sexual activity, painful intercourse, diminished sexual responsiveness, difficulty achieving orgasm, and decreased genital sensation. The decrease in serum estrogen levels results in thinning of the vaginal mucosal epithelium, atrophy of vaginal wall smooth muscle and change in vaginal pH. These changes may lead to vaginal infections, urinary tract infections, and incontinence, and complaints of sexual dysfunction [74]. Older women and menopausal women not receiving hormone replacement therapy have decreased genital blood flow when compared with controls [75]. Immunohistochemical studies in human vaginal tissues have revealed the presence of nerve fibers containing neuropeptide Y, vasoactive intestinal polypeptide (VIP), NOS, cGMP and substance P [76, 77]. NO has been identified in the clitoris of women and has been proposed to be the primary mediator of clitoral and labial engorgement [78, 79]. We have shown in our laboratory that the rat clitoris and vagina contain these neurotransmitters. Furthermore, we have demonstrated that the vaginal and clitoral blood flow are sensitive to neuropressors such as NO donors in the female rat [Carrier et al., 2003, unpubl. data]. Aging and surgical castration result in decreased vaginal and clitoral NOS expression. Estrogen replacement restores vaginal mucosal health, increases vaginal NOS expression, and decreases vaginal mucosal cell death [80]. The different phases of the sexual cycle, as well as their physiological control, are similar in human males and females [81]. In women, this decrease in neurotransmitter will have an impact on the sexual arousal phase and lead to a decreased vaginal lubrication, making sexual intercourse unpleasant. Sensory thresholds in the pudendal nerve seem to be affected by the level of circulating estradiol as suggested by animal models. Estrogen replacement restores clitoral and vaginal vibration and pressure thresholds in postmenopausal women to levels close to the levels in premenopausal women [74]. Testosterone levels also decrease in older women and these changes have been associated with a decline in sexual arousal, genital sensation, libido, and orgasm [82]. Initial therapeutic success using testosterone for inhibited desire in naturally menopausal women has been reported.

Finally, it should be noted that although ovarian production of estrogens ceases with a natural or surgical menopause, cross-sectional studies indicate that serum estrogen levels vary greatly in older postmenopausal women not receiving hormonal replacement [83]. Studies indicate nonovarian cells, particularly those in adipose tissues continue to convert adrenal precursors to low-potency estrogens [84]. As a result, levels of endogenous estrogens correlate more strongly with body mass index than with age or time from menopause [83]. In recent years, increasing attention has been paid to these endogenous estrogens since they appear to influence the development of bone loss and fractures in older women [84, 85], although the impact of these hormones on other estrogen-responsive tissues such as the reproductive tissues remains to be established.

References

1   Sauer MV: The impact of age on reproductive potential: Lesson learned from oocyte donation. Maturitas 1998;30:221–225.
2   Fitzgerald C, Zimon AE, Jones EE: Aging and reproductive potential in women. Yale J Biol Med 1998;71:367–381.
3   Levran D, Ben-Shlomo I, Dor J, Ben-Rafael Z, Nevel L, Mashiach S: Aging of endometrium and oocytes: Observation on conception an abortion rates in an egg donation model. Fertil Steril 1991;56:1901–1904.
4   Navot D, Bergh PA, William MA, Garrisi GJ, Guzman I, Sandler B, Grunfeld L: Poor oocyte quality rather than implantation failure as a cause of age-related decline in female fertility. Lancet 1991;337:1375–1377.
5   Tietze C: Reproductive span and rate of reproduction among Hutterite women. Fertil Steril 1957; 8:89–97.
6   Craft I, Ah-Moye M, Al-Shawaf T, Fiamanya W, Lewis P, Robertson D, Serhal P, Shrivastav P, Simons E, Brinsden P: Analysis of 1071 GIFT procedures – The case for flexible a approach to treatment. Lancet 1988;i:1094–1097.
7   Beral V, Doyle P, Tan SL, Mason BA, Campbell S: Outcome of pregnancies resulting from assisted conception. Br Med Bull 1990;46:769–782.
8   Al-Shawaf T, Nolan A, Guirgis R, Harper J, Santis M, Craft I: The influence of ovarian response on gamete intra-Fallopian transfer outcome in older women. Hum Reprod 1992;7:1106–1110.
9   Schwartz D, Mayaux MJ: Female fecundity as a function of age: Results of artificial insemination in 2,193 nulliparous women with azoospermic husbands. N Engl J Med 1982;306:404–406.
10   Shenfield F, Doyle P, Valentine A, Steele SJ, Tan SL: Effect of age, gravidity and male infertility status in cumulative conception rates following artificial insemination with cryopreserved donor semen: Analysis of 2,998 cycles of treatment in one centre over 10 years. Hum Reprod 1993;8:60–64.
11   Stovall DW, Toma SK, Hammond MG, Talbert LM: The effect of age on female fecundity. Obstet Gynecol 1991;77:33–36.
12   Wang AW, Ho PC, Kwan M, Ma HK: Factors affecting the success of artificial insemination by frozen donor semen. Int J Fertil 1989;34:25–29.
13   Tan SL, Royston P, Campbell S, Jacobs HS, Betts J, Mason B, Edwards RG: Cumulative conception and livebirth rates after in-vitro fertilization. Lancet 1992;339:1390–1394.
14   Piette C, Mouzon J, Bachelot A, Spira A: In-vitro fertilization: Influence of women's age on pregnancy rates. Hum Reprod 1990;5:56–59.
15   Wood C, Calderon I, Crombie A: Age and fertility: Results of assisted reproductive technology in women over 40 years. J Assist Reprod Genet 1992;9:482–484.
16   Harrison KL, Breen TM, Hennessey JF, Hynes MJ, Keeping JD, Kilvert GT, DeAmbrosis PJ, Molloy D: Patient age and the success in a human IVF programme. Aust NZ J Obstet Gynaecol 1989;29:326–328.

17   Lau WNT, So WWK, Yeung WSB, Ho PC: The effect of aging on female fertility in an assisted reproduction programme in Hong Kong: Retrospective study. Hong Kong Med J 2000;6:147–152.
18   Hermann M, Berger P: Aging of the male endocrine system. Rev Physiol Biochem Pharmacol 1999;139:90–122.
19   Neaves WB, Johnson L, Porter JC, Panker CR Jr, Petty CS: Leydig cell numbers, daily sperm production and serum gonadotropin levels in aging men. J Clin Endocr Metab 1984;59:759–763.
20   Johnson L, Petty CS, Neaves WB: Influence of age on sperm production and testicular weight in men. J Reprod Fertil 1984;70:211–218.
21   Holstein AF: Human spermatogenesis in old age, a borderland between normal and pathological anatomy. Urologe A 1986;25:130–137.
22   Vermiulen A: Biological manifestations of the andropause. Fiziol Zh 1990;36:90–93.
23   Fukuda T, Kikuchi M, Kurotaki T, Oyamada T, Yoshikawa H, Yoshikawa T: Age-related changes in the testes of horses. Equine Vet J 2001;33:20–25.
24   Rolf C, Behre HM, Nieschlag E: Reproductive parameters of older compared to young men of infertile couples. Int J Androl 1996;19:135–142.
25   Spandorfer SD, Avrech OM, Colombero LT, Palermo GD, Rosenwaks Z: Effect of parental age on fertilization and pregnancy characteristics in couples treated by intracytoplasmic sperm injection. Hum Reprod 1998;13:334–338.
26   Pals E, Berger P, Hermann M, Pfluger H: Effect of aging on male fertility. Exp Gerontol 2000; 35:543–551.
27   Schwartz D, Mayaux MJ, Spria A, Moscato ML, Jouannet P, Czyglik F, David G: Semen characteristics as a function of age in 833 fertile men. Fertil Steril 1983;39:530–535.
28   Nieschlag E, Lammers U, Freischem CW, Langer K, Wicking EJ: Reproductive functions in young fathers and grandfathers. J Clin Endocr Metab 1982;55:676–681.
29   Check JH, Shanis B, Bollendrof A, Adelson H, Breen E: Semen characteristics and infertility in aging. Arch Androl 1989;23:275–277.
30   Meacham RB, Murray MJ: Reproductive function in aging male. Urol Clin North Am 1994;21: 549–556.
31   Haidl G, Jung A, Schill WB: Aging and sperm function. Hum Reprod 1996;11:558–560.
32   Liam JH, Zack MM, Erickson JD: Paternal age and the occurrence of birth defects. Am J Hum Genet 1986;39:648–660.
33   Friedman JM: Genetic disease in the offspring of older father. Obstet Gynecol 1981;57:745–749.
34   Risch N, Reich EW, Wishnick MM, McCarthy JG: Spontaneous mutation and parental age in human. Am J Hum Genet 1987;41:218–248.
35   Bordson BL, Leonardo VS: The appropriate upper age limit for several semen donors: A review of the genetic effects of the paternal age. Fertil Steril 1991;56:397–401.
36   Morales A, Heaton JPW, Carson CC: Andropause: A misnomer for a true clinical entity. J Urol 2000;163:705–712.
37   Vermeulen A, Kaufman JM: Aging of the hypothalamo-pituitary-testicular axis in men. Horm Res 1995;43:25–32.
38   Lamberts SW, van den Beld AW, van der Lely AJ: The endocrinology of aging. Science 1997;278: 419–424.
39   Johannes CB, Araujo AB, Feldman HA, Derby CA, Kleinman KP, McKinlay JB: Incidence of erectile dysfunction in men 40 to 69 years old: Longitudinal results from the Massachusetts male aging study. J Urol 2000;163:460–463.
40   Helgason AR, Adolfsson J, Dickman P, Arver S, Fredrikson M, Gothberg M, Steineck G: Sexual desire, erection, orgasm and ejaculatory functions and their importance to elderly Swedish men: A population-based study. Age Ageing 1996;25:285–291.
41   Schill WB: Fertility and sexual life of men after their forties and in older age. Asian J Androl 2001;3:1–7.
42   Wespes E: Erectile dysfunction in the ageing man. Curr Opin Urol 2000;10:625–628.
43   Calcaterra R, Cembalo G, Belmonte M, Merante A, Mattace R: Sexuality of elderly women. Minerva Med 1996;87:311–315.
44   Hsueh W: Sexual dysfunction with aging and systemic hypertension. Am J Cardiol 1988;61:18–23.
45   Quadri R, Fonzo D: Libido-related changes in the elderly. Arch Ital Urol Androl 1993;65:487–489.

46   Clark JT: Sexual function in altered physiological states: Comparison of effects of hypertension, diabetes, hyperprolactinemia, and others to 'normal' aging in male rats. Neurosci Biobehav Rev 1995;19:279–302.

47   Calabro A, Italiano G, Pescatori ES, Marin A, Gaetano O, Abatangelo G, Pagano F: Physiological aging and penile erectile function: A study in the rat. Eur Urol 1996;29:240–244.

48   Meston CM: Aging and sexuality. West J Med 1997;167:285–290.

49   Aresin L: Sexual behavior in higher age. Z Gesamte Inn Med 1976;31:120–123.

50   Kidd SA, Eskenazi B, Wyrobek AJ: Effects of male age on semen quality and fertility: A review of the literature. Fertil Steril 2001;75:237–248.

51   Segraves RT: Antidepressant-induced orgasm disorder. J Sex Marital Ther 1995;21:192–201.

52   Akkus E, Carrier S, Baba K, Hsu GL, Padma-Nathan H, Nunes L, Lue TF: Structural alterations in the tunica albuginea of the penis: Impact of Peyronie's disease, ageing and impotence. Br J Urol 1997;79:47–53.

53   Higami Y, Shimokawa I: Apoptosis in the aging process. Cell Tissue Res 2000;301:125–132.

54   Carrier S, Nagaraju P, Morgan DM, Baba K, Nunes L, Lue TF: Age decreases nitric oxide synthase-containing nerve fibers in the rat penis. J Urol 1997;157:1088–1092.

55   Dahiya R, Chui R, Perinchery G, Nakajima K, Oh BR, Lue TF: Differential gene expression of growth factors in young and old rat penile tissues is associated with erectile dysfunction. Int J Impot Res 1999;11:201–206.

56   Jiaan DB, Seftel AD, Fogarty J, Hampel N, Cruz W, Pomerantz J, Zuik M, Monnier VM: Age-related increase in an advanced glycation end product in penile tissue. World J Urol 1995;13: 369–375.

57   Baba K, Yajima M, Carrier S, Akkus E, Reman J, Nunes L, Lue TF, Iwamoto T: Effect of testosterone on the number of NADPH diaphorase-stained nerve fibers in the rat corpus cavernosum and dorsal nerve. Urology 2000;56:533–538.

58   Baba K, Yajima M, Carrier S, Morgan DM, Nunes L, Lue TF, Iwamoto T: Delayed testosterone replacement restores nitric oxide synthase-containing nerve fibres and the erectile response in rat penis. BJU Int 2000;85:953–958.

59   Schochet SS: Neuropathology of aging. Neurol Clin 1998;16:569–580.

60   Bemelmans BL, Meuleman EJ, Anten BW, Doesburg WH, Van Kerrebroeck PE, Debruyne FM: Penile sensory disorders in erectile dysfunction: Results of a comprehensive neuro-urophysiological diagnostic evaluation in 123 patients. J Urol 1991;146:777–782.

61   Pfeifer J, Salanga VD, Agachan F, Weiss EG, Wexner SD: Variation in pudendal nerve terminal motor latency according to disease. Dis Colon Rectum 1997;40:79–83.

62   Jameson JS, Chia YW, Kamm MA, Speakman CT, Chye YH, Henry M: Effect of age, sex and parity on anorectal function. Br J Surg 1994;81:1689–1692.

63   Lefaucheur J, Yiou R, Thomas C: Pudendal nerve terminal motor latency: Age effects and technical considerations. Clin Neurophysiol 2001;112:472–476.

64   Johnson RD, Murray FT: Reduced sensitivity of penile mechanoreceptors in aging rats with sexual dysfunction. Brain Res Bull 1992;28:61–64.

65   Schmidt RE, Dorsey DA, McDaniel ML, Corbett JA: Characterization of NADPH diaphorase activity in rat sympathetic autonomic ganglia – Effect of diabetes and aging. Brain Res 1993;617: 343–348.

66   Ackerman AE, Lange GM, Clemens LG: Effects of paraventricular lesions on sex behavior and seminal emission in male rats. Physiol Behav 1997;63:49–53.

67   Arletti R, Benelli A, Bertolini A: Sexual behavior of aging male rats is stimulated by oxytocin. Eur J Pharmacol 1990;179:377–381.

68   Hung SH, Pi WP, Tsai YF, Peng MT: Restoration of sexual behavior in aged male rats by intracerebral grafts of fetal preoptic area neurons. J Formos Med Assoc 1997;96:812–818.

69   Liu M, Chino N, Takahashi H: Current status of rehabilitation, especially in-patients with stroke, in Japan. Scand J Rehabil Med 2000;32:148–158.

70   Marinkovic S, Badlani G: Voiding and sexual dysfunction after cerebrovascular accidents. J Urol 2001;165:359–370.

71   Coslett HB, Heilman KM: Male sexual function. Impairment after right hemisphere stroke. Arch Neurol 1986;43:1036–1039.

72   Kaiser FE: Sexuality in the elderly. Urol Clin North Am 1996;23:99–109.
73   Alexander CJ, Sipski ML, Findley TW: Sexual activities, desire, and satisfaction in males pre- and post-spinal cord injury. Arch Sex Behav 1993;22:217–228.
74   Sarrell PM: Sexuality and menopause. Obstet Gynecol 1990;75:26s.
75   Carlson KJ: Outcomes of hysterectomy. Clin Obstet Gynecol 1997;40:939–946.
76   Hoyle CH, Stones RW, Robson T, Whitley K, Burnstock G: Innervation of vasculature and microvasculature of human vagina by NOS and neuropeptide-containing nerves. J Anat 1996;188: 633–644.
77   Hsueh WA: Sexual dysfunction with aging and systemic hypertension. Am J Cardiol 1998;61: 18H–23H.
78   Burnett AL, Calvin DC, Silver RI, Peppas DS, Docimo SG: Immunohistochemical description of nitric oxide synthase isoforms in human clitoris. J Urology 1997;158:75–78.
79   Park K, Moreland RB, Goldstein I, Atala A, Traish A: Characterization of phosphodiesterase activity in human clitoral corpus cavernosum smooth muscle cells in culture. Biochem Biophys Res Commun 1998;249:612–617.
80   Berman JR, Berman L, Goldstein I: Female sexual dysfunction: Incidence, pathophysiology, evaluation, and treatment options. Urology 1999;54:385–391.
81   Berman JR, Goldstein I: Female sexual dysfunction. Urol Clin North Am 2000;28:405–416.
82   Davis SR: Androgens and female sexuality. J Gender Specific Med 2000;3:36–40.
83   Meldrum DR, Davidson BJ, Tataryn IV, Judd HL: Changes in circulating steroids with aging in postmenopausal women. Obstet Gynecol 1981;57:624–628.
84   Kuchel GA, Tannenbaum C, Greenspan SL, Resnick NM: Can variability in the hormonal status of elderly women assist in the decision to administer estrogens? J Womens Health Gend Based Med 2001;10:109–116.
85   Cummings SR, Browner WS, Bauer D, Stone K, Ensrud K, Jamal S, Ettinger B: Endogenous hormones and the risk of hip and vertebral fractures among older women. Study of Osteoporotic Fractures Research Group. N Engl J Med 1998;339:733–738.

Serge Carrier, MD, FRCS(C)
687 Pine Avenue West
Royal Victoria Hospital S6.92, Montreal, Quebec, H3A 1A1 (Canada)
Tel. +1 514 842 1231 X34302, Fax +1 514 843 1552, E-Mail serge.carrier@mcgill.ca

Kuchel GA, Hof PR (eds): Autonomic Nervous System in Old Age.
Interdiscipl Top Gerontol. Basel, Karger, 2004, vol 33, pp 107–119

....

Aging of the Autonomic Nervous System

Pain Perception

David Lussier[a,b]*, Ricardo A. Cruciani*[b]

[a] Division of Geriatric Medicine, McGill University, Montreal, Quebec, Canada,
[b] Department of Pain Medicine and Palliative Care, Beth Israel Medical Center,
New York, N.Y., USA

Pain is a multidimensional experience, defined as 'an unpleasant sensory and emotional experience associated with actual or potential tissue damage, or described in terms of such damage' [1]. Pain is therefore a subjective experience, distinct from nociception ('detection of tissue damage by specialized transducers attached to A delta and C fibres') [2], which represents the anatomical and physiological components of pain.

There is currently no consensus on the role of the autonomic nervous system (ANS) in pain perception, nor on age-related changes in ANS or pain perception. The implications of the age-related ANS changes on pain perception are even less clear. In this chapter, we will review experimental data from animal and human studies that can contribute to a better understanding of this important area of pain pathophysiology.

Epidemiology of Pain in Old Age

Pain is a frequent complaint in older persons. The prevalence of persistent (or 'chronic') pain in community-dwelling older persons ranges between 40 and 75%, depending on the population studied and the definition of persistent pain [3–7]. It seems to be more frequent among the oldest old and among women [3–5]. Pain is also the symptom most frequently reported by community-dwelling elderly individuals (73%) [8].

Pain Perception in Older Persons

The subjective nature of pain renders its study difficult, as there is no reliable objective measure of pain intensity. Most data on this topic are based on acute experimental pain. Unfortunately, the relevance of acute experimental pain to clinical pain is unclear, as is that of animal studies. Moreover, even though experimental pain is less subject to psychological influences than clinical pain, the person's pain detection and tolerance thresholds are still modulated by these factors, which makes it impossible to attribute observed differences to the sole effect of physiological changes [9].

Pain detection threshold ('the lowest value at which the person reports that the stimulation feels painful' [10]) is the most objective indicator of pain perception. An age-related increase in the detection threshold for cutaneous thermal pain [11–15] and cutaneous electric current [16, 17] has been reported. However, the results have been conflicting [18], with evidence of considerable intersubject variability in the oldest old [17].

As pain tolerance ('the value at which the subject withdraws or asks to have the stimulation stopped' [10]) is more affected by cognitive appraisals of the pain stimulation than is pain detection threshold, it is even more subject to inter-individual variability. The rare studies on age-related changes in pain tolerance point towards a possible decreased tolerance [19–21].

Overall, the conflicting and variable results of these studies have led Harkins [22] to conclude from his review that 'effects of aging on pain are less important than the effects of pain on successful aging'.

Physiologic Basis of Pain Perception

A discussion of the physiologic basis of pain perception is beyond the scope of this chapter and the reader is referred to several detailed reviews of this topic [23–26].

Pain perception is the result of interactions between the peripheral nervous system, the central nervous system (ascending and descending pathways, brain), intrinsic neural inhibitory modulation and the activity of the body's stress-regulation systems (including endocrine, autonomic, immune and opioid systems as well as cytokines) (fig. 1) [27].

Nociceptors are peripheral endings of primary sensory neurons, which are located in skin, muscles, fascia, blood vessels walls, tendons, joint capsules, ligaments, fat pads and periosteum [28]. The activation of these nociceptors results in noxious afferent impulses, which are then transmitted through Aδ and C fibers [23].

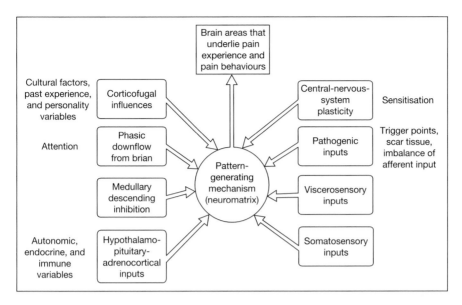

Fig. 1. Pattern-generating mechanism or neuromatrix modulated by multiple inputs and the internal milieu. Pain perception is the result of interactions between the peripheral nervous system, the central nervous system, intrinsic neural inhibitory modulation and the activity of the body's stress-regulation systems. The neuromatrix model integrates all these components. Reproduced with permission from Loeser and Melzack [2].

The Aδ fibers are large-caliber, thinly myelinated, fast-conducting fibers responsible for the transmission of epicritic or phasic pain ('first pain'), evoking pain described as pricking, sharp and well localized [25]. C fibers are polymodal, slow-conducting nonmyelinated fibers that respond to mechanical, heat and chemical stimuli [25]. Due to their larger receptive fields ($100 \, mm^2$ in humans) [28], they transmit poorly localized pain sensations, often described as dull and burning, and referred to as tonic pain, or 'second pain'.

At the spinal cord level, primary afferent nociceptive fibers terminate primarily in the superficial dorsal horn in lamina I (marginal zone) and lamina II (substantia gelatinosa). Lamina V projection neurons also receive input from Aδ fibers [26].

The nociceptive information is then transmitted to the brain along five major ascending pathways: the spinothalamic, spinoreticular, spinomesencephalic and spinocervical tracts, as well as the dorsal columns of the spinal cord (fig. 2) [26]. These pathways all project to the mesencephalon and the diencephalon [23]. Multiple brain areas are involved in the central representation of pain, including the thalamus, the primary and secondary somatosensory areas of the

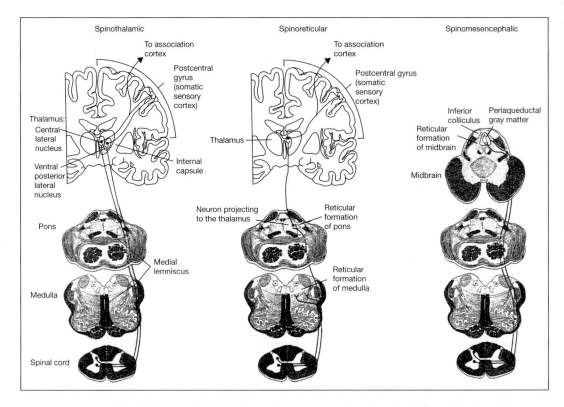

Fig. 2. Three major ascending pathways transmit nociceptive information from the dorsal horn of the spinal cord to the mesencephalon and the diencephalon: the spinothalamic, the spinoreticular and the spinomesencephalic tracts. The spinocervical tract and the dorsal columns of the spinal cord, also involved in transmission of nociception, are not represented here. Reproduced with permission from Jessell and Kelly [26].

cerebral cortex, the anterior cingulate cortex, the anterior insula, the prefrontal cortex and the posterior parietal cortex [29]. These regions form a neural network, with components sub serving the different dimensions of the pain experience [27].

Neurons present within these brain regions have been found to exert a bi-directional control over dorsal horn nociceptive transmission neurons [30]. Several central mechanisms are involved in the modulation of pain, including a descending inhibitory pathway that originates from the midbrain and makes excitatory connections in the rostroventral medulla, from where projection neurons make inhibitory connections in the dorsal horn [26, 30]. Central opioid receptors present in these neurons are activated both by endogenous opioid peptides (endorphins) and exogenous opioids, which produce analgesia by activating the descending pain modulatory pathways [30]. These endogenous pain-inhibitory systems can also be activated by nociceptive or stressful stimuli [26, 30, 31] and can be classified as nonhormonal/opioid (e.g. electric shock), hormonal/opioid (e.g. food deprivation), nonhormonal/nonopioid (e.g. neural, ex. repetitive stimulation of Aβ sensory fibers) and hormonal/nonopioid (e.g. cold pressor test, cold water immersion) [32]. However, under conditions of severe environmental stress or high-intensity ongoing noxious input, all inhibitory systems are activated [30].

Several chemicals (bradykinin, histamine, serotonin, prostaglandins) and peptides (substance P, GABA, calcitonin) are involved in the neurotransmission of nociception at the supraspinal and spinal levels [23].

Role of the Autonomic Nervous System in Nociception

Under normal physiologic circumstances, the role of the ANS resides mainly in the supraspinal modulation of nociception. Norepinephrine is the neurotransmitter of a major descending inhibitory pathway and is crucial in the analgesic actions of systemically administered opioids. Analgesia also results from direct application of norepinephrine to the spinal cord [26]. Studies using the partial agonist clonidine and the antagonist yohimbine have shown that activation of the α_2-adrenergic receptors located on the brainstem projections results in a decrease in substance P release [33, 34] and of wide dynamic range neuron discharge [35]. In contrast, the activation of α_1-adrenergic receptors has no effect [33, 35]. Clonidine has strong antinociceptive effects in animals [36] and is effective in relieving diverse pain syndromes in a subset of human patients when administered intraspinally or systemically [37–39]. Inhibition of spinal cholinesterase produces an acute dose-dependent analgesic response [40, 41] which is antagonized by muscarinic antagonists [42] whereas muscarinic agonists are antinociceptive [43].

The ANS is also involved in the physiological responses (tachycardia, tachypnea) and protective reactions associated with pain [44].

Its role is pivotal in the generation of some pathological pain syndromes, of which complex regional pain syndrome type I (causalgia) and type II (reflex sympathetic dystrophy) and other neuropathic pain syndromes (postherpetic neuralgia, painful metabolic neuropathies, phantom pain, traumatic nerve injury) are the most common [45]. In some of these syndromes, classified as 'sympathetically maintained', nociceptors are excited and possibly sensitized by norepinephrine released by sympathetic fibers, either directly (via adreno-receptors located in the nociceptors) or indirectly (via the vascular bed).

This then generates a state of central sensitization/hyperexcitability leading to spontaneous pain and allodynia (pain evoked by a nonnoxious stimulus) [44]. Blockade of the sympathetic activity can sometimes be beneficial.

Mechanisms of Age-Related Changes in Nociception

Age-related changes in the pain experience include changes in the perception, transmission and modulation of nociception. Figure 3 illustrates the known and potential effects of aging on pain systems.

Peripheral Nervous System
Several studies point to a role of the peripheral nervous system in the age-related changes of nociception. Chakour et al. [15] found some evidence for a differential aging of Aδ and C-fibers by studying the effect on CO_2 laser-induced thermal pain thresholds of an A-fiber specific block of the superficial radial nerve. Whereas older subjects' pain threshold was higher than their younger counterparts' before and after the block, the thresholds of the two age groups were similar during the block, due to increased thresholds in both groups but of much greater magnitude in the younger group. Similarly, Harkins et al. [46] observed delayed response times to first pain in older subjects, without modification of response times to second pain. These studies suggest that a selective age-related alteration in Aδ fibers, which are responsible for the epicritic pain perception, might partly account for the changes in nociception observed with aging, more specifically the delayed pain perception and the less precise description and localization of pain sensations.

Age-related impairments have also been reported for C fibers, including decreased conduction and function [47–49], as well as for C-fiber-mediated sensitization of second-order nociceptive neurons, as suggested by the absence of slow temporal summation of second pain following repeated thermal stimulation of the legs in older subjects [46].

Central Nervous System
According to animal studies, the opioidergic system undergoes several changes with aging [50]. The concentration of opioid receptors in the brain decreases [51], but the binding affinity of the opioids for their receptors does not seem to be modified [52]. The concentration of endogenous opioids in the dorsal horn is decreased at some levels of the spinal cord [53], accompanied by a decrease in levels of circulating β-endorphins [54, 55]. The analgesic response following the administration of morphine and other μ-receptor agonists is reduced [56], while the response to exogenous β-endorphins is preserved [57],

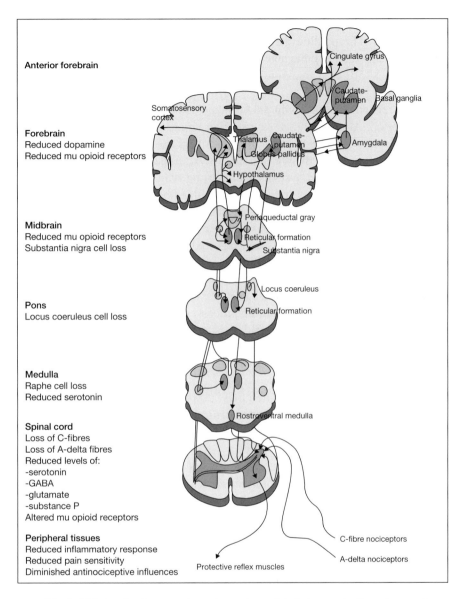

Anterior forebrain

Cingulate gyrus

Caudate-putamen Basal ganglia

Somatosensory cortex

Forebrain
Reduced dopamine
Reduced mu opioid receptors

Thalamus Caudate-putamen

Globus pallidus

Amygdala

Hypothalamus

Midbrain
Reduced mu opioid receptors
Substantia nigra cell loss

Periaqueductal gray

Reticular formation

Substantia nigra

Pons
Locus coeruleus cell loss

Locus coeruleus

Reticular formation

Medulla
Raphe cell loss
Reduced serotonin

Spinal cord
Loss of C-fibres
Loss of A-delta fibres
Reduced levels of:
-serotonin
-GABA
-glutamate
-substance P
Altered mu opioid receptors

Rostroventral medulla

Peripheral tissues
Reduced inflammatory response
Reduced pain sensitivity
Diminished antinociceptive influences

C-fibre nociceptors

A-delta nociceptors

Protective reflex muscles

Fig. 3. Effects of aging on pain systems. Age-related changes in the pain experience occur at each level of the perception, transmission and modulation of nociception. Some of the changes described in this figure have however not been observed consistently in humans. Reproduced with permission from Franklin and Abbott [79].

suggesting a variability in the age-related changes in the response to opioid agonists [58]. The opioid-mediated pain-inhibitory descending pathway also seems to be altered [59]. None of these findings has however been observed in older humans [50], in whom opioid agonist drugs are as effective as in younger people [60].

Age-related decrements in other endogenous analgesic systems have also been reported. Animal studies suggest that aging might be associated with a general decline in neurally mediated nonopioid pain-inhibitory systems activated by noxious or stressful stimuli [58, 61, 62], whereas the senescence of the hormonally mediated systems seems to be more complex [63]. A similar decline seems to be present in humans as well. Although present, the analgesic response following cold water immersion of the hand is of much lower magnitude in older compared to younger volunteers [31]. Facilitation of thermal pain, rather than inhibition, has even been reported using a similar procedure [64]. Together, these results suggest that aging might be associated with an impairment of some endogenous pain-modulatory systems, which might contribute to the high prevalence of pain in the elderly.

Age-related changes of the brain processes of pain have also been demonstrated. The electroencephalographic response to a nociceptive stimulation is delayed and of smaller amplitude, as well as more widespread and less specific [65].

Age-Related Changes of Autonomic Nervous System-Mediated Pain

As stated above, one of the major descending pain inhibitory pathways is mediated, at least in part, by the muscarinic cholinergic system [66]. According to animal studies, aging is associated with a general decline of the cholinergic system, including decreases in the density of muscarinic and nicotinic receptor-binding sites [51, 67]. Unexpectedly, the endogenous pain inhibition system of aged animals, however, remains sensitive or becomes hypersensitive to the stimulation of the postsynaptic cholinergic receptor by the muscarinic cholinergic agonist oxotremorine [68, 69] or the increased presynaptic level of acetylcholine by the anticholinesterase agent physostigmine [67]. The analgesic response to the α_2-adrenergic agonist clonidine is not modified either [70]. In contrast, there is an attenuation of the ability of the muscarinic cholinergic antagonist scopolamine to attenuate the analgesia produced by electric shocks, and a general decline in the activity of the endogenous, cholinergically mediated pain-inhibitory descending pathway [71]. This might suggest that the age-related decline in the endogenous analgesia function is the result of a deficit in the presynaptic release of acetylcholine rather than a decline in a postsynaptic process, and that aging is accompanied by a compensating alteration in the dynamics of the cholinergic receptor function that mediates the analgesic response [67]. Several other factors and biases may, however, also account for these observations [50]. None of these studies has been replicated in humans, but an enhanced acute increase in norepinephrine following a cold pressor test has been reported in subjects older than 80 years old [72]. Furthermore, although it has not been studied specifically, clinical experience does not suggest any difference in the analgesic response to clonidine in older patients.

There is currently no evidence in the literature indicating that the prevalence of sympathetically maintained pain in the elderly differs from the general population. Due to the overall increase in pain prevalence with age, sympathetically maintained pain could actually be more frequent in the elderly [73]. Following partial nerve injury (e.g. post-herpetic neuralgia), older patients are more likely than younger patients to develop persistent pain [74].

Conflicting results have been reported on the age-related changes of partial nerve injury-induced neuropathic pain in animals. The very few studies conducted on this topic showed either increased [75] or decreased [76] behavioral responses to nerve ligation in rats. Older rats often fail to develop allodynia in these circumstances [77].

Ramer and Bisby [73] reported that sympathetic innervation of rat dorsal root ganglion (DRG) naturally increases with age and that older rats have more nocifensive behaviors in response to thermal and mechanical stimulation. The explanations of these phenomena are currently unclear [73].

Ramer and Bisby [73] also observed that sympathetic-fiber density following chronic sciatic nerve constriction injury was greater in old (16 months old) than in young (3 months old) rats. Thermal hyperalgesia and mechanical allodynia were more pronounced in old rats and, in another study, have been shown to be correlated with sympathetic sprouting in the DRG [78]. This sprouting could therefore be responsible for the sympathetic generation or maintenance of pain. The increased sympathetic innervation observed in noninjured animals, if it also occurs in humans, could partly explain the increased prevalence of neuropathic and sympathetically maintained pain in the elderly [50].

Conclusion

Persistent pain is a frequent problem in older people. Although studies on age-related changes in experimental pain perception have reported inconsistent results, there seems to be an increase in the pain detection threshold to some nociceptive stimuli. These changes are explained by alterations in the peripheral and central nervous systems, including a selective impairment of Aδ-fibers and an attenuation of some endogenous descending pain-inhibitory pathways.

The ANS is mainly involved in the supraspinal modulation of pain perception, which partly relies on a cholinergically mediated pain-inhibitory pathway. Age-related changes in this system reported in animal studies might contribute to the increased prevalence of pain in older persons. An increase in sympathetic sprouting of the dorsal root ganglion associated with aging observed in non-injured animals, as well as increased sympathetic sprouting following chronic constriction injury, might predispose older patients to the development of chronic neuropathic and sympathetically maintained pain following partial nerve injury. However, there is currently no such findings in humans and it is unclear whether results from these animal studies can be applied to humans.

Hopefully, future studies will provide a better knowledge of the age-related changes in nociception, which would allow the development of new therapeutic strategies to improve the pain relief in older patients.

Acknowledgement

We would like to thank Mark Bisby for criticism and advice on an early version of this chapter.

References

1   Merskey H: Classification of chronic pain: Descriptions of chronic pain syndromes and defini-
    tions of pain terms. Pain 1986;(suppl 3):S1–S222.
2   Loeser JD, Melzack R: Pain: An overview. Lancet 1999;353:1607–1609.
3   Brattberg G, Parker MG, Thorslund M: The prevalence of pain among the oldest old in Sweden.
    Pain 1996;67:29–34.
4   Brochet B, Michel P, Barberger-Gateau P, Dartigues JF: Population-based study of pain in elderly
    people: A descriptive survey. Age Ageing 1998;27:279–284.
5   Elliott AM, Smith BH, Penny KI, Smith WC, Chambers WA: The epidemiology of chronic pain
    in the community. Lancet 1999;354:1248–1252.
6   Landi F, Onder G, Cesari M, Gambassi G, Steel K, Russo A, Lattanzio F, Bernabei R: The epidemi-
    ology of chronic pain in the community. Arch Intern Med 2001;161:2731–2734.
7   Ross MM, Crook J: Elderly recipients of home nursing services: Pain, disability and functional
    competence. J Adv Nurs 1998;27:1117–1126.
8   Brody EM, Kleban MH: Day-to-day mental and physical health symptoms of older people: A report
    on health logs. Gerontologist 1983;23:75–85.
9   Harkins SW: Geriatric pain: Pain perceptions in the old. Clin Geriatr Med 1996;12:435–459.
10 Melzack R, Wall PD: The Challenge of Pain. London, Penguin Books, 1988.
11 Sherman ED, Robillard E: Sensitivity to pain in the aged. CMAJ 1960;38:944–947.
12 Schludermann E, Zubek JP: Effect of age on pain sensitivity. Percept Motor Skills 1962;14:295–301.
13 Procacci P, Bozza G, Buzzelli G, Della Corte M: The cutaneous pricking pain threshold in old age.
    Gerontol Clin 1970;12:213–218.

14   Gibson SJ, Gorman MM, Helme RD: Assessment of pain in the elderly using event-related cerebral potentials; in Bond MR, Charlton JE, Woolf CJ (eds): Proceedings of the VIth World Congress on Pain. New York, Elsevier, 1991, pp 527–533.

15   Chakour MC, Gibson SJ, Bradbeer M, Helme RD: The effect of age on A delta and C-fibre thermal pain perception. Pain 1996;64:143–152.

16   Neri M, Agazzani E: Aging and right-left asymmetry in experimental pain measurement. Pain 1984;19:43–48.

17   Tucker MA, Andrew MF, Ogle SJ, Davison JG: Age-associated change in pain threshold measured by transcutaneous neuronal electrical stimulation. Age Ageing 1989;18:241–246.

18   Kenshalo DR: Somesthetic sensitivity in young and elderly humans. J Gerontol 1986;41:732–742.

19   Collins LG, Stone LA: Pain sensitivity, age and activity level in chronic schizophrenics and in normals. Br J Psychol 1966;112:33–35.

20   Walsh NE, Schoenfeld L, Ramamurthy S, Hoffman J: Normative model for cold pressor test. Am J Phys Med Rehabil 1989;68:6–11.

21   Woodrow KM, Friedman GD, Siegelaub AB, Collen MF: Pain tolerance: Differences according to age, sex and race. Psychosom Med 1972;34:548–556.

22   Harkins WS: What is unique about the older adult's pain experience? in Weiner DK, Herr K, Rudy TE (eds): Persistent Pain in Older Adults: An Interdisciplinary Guide for Treatment. New York, Springer, 2002, pp 4–17.

23   Besson JM: The neurobiology of pain. Lancet 1999;353:1610–1615.

24   Markenson JA: Mechanisms of chronic pain. Am J Med 1996;101(suppl 1A):6S–18S.

25   Raja SN, Meyer RA, Ringkamp M, Campbell JN: Peripheral neural mechanisms of nociception; in Wall PD, Melzack R (eds): Textbook of Pain, ed 4. New York, Churchill Livingstone, 1999, pp 11–58.

26   Jessell TM, Kelly DD: Pain and analgesia; in Kandel ER, Schwartz JH, Jessell TM (eds): Principles of Neural Science, ed 3. Norwalk, Appleton & Lange, 1991, pp 385–399.

27   Melzack R: From the gate to the neuromatrix. Pain 1999;(suppl 6):S121–S126.

28   Schmidt R, Schmelz M, Ringkamp M, Handwerker HO, Torebjork HE: Innervation territories of mechanically activated C nociceptor units in human skin. J Neurophysiology 1997;78:2641–2648.

29   Ingvar M, Hsieh JC: The image of pain; in Wall PD, Melzack R (eds): Textbook of Pain, ed 4. New York, Churchill Livingstone, 1999, pp 215–234.

30   Fields HL, Basbaum AI: Central nervous system mechanisms of pain modulation; in Wall PD, Melzack R (eds): Textbook of Pain, ed 4. New York, Churchill Livingstone, 1999, pp 309–329.

31   Washington LL, Gibson SJ, Helme RD: Age-related differences in the endogenous analgesic response to repeated cold water immersion in human volunteers. Pain 2000;89:89–96.

32   Watkins LR, Mayer DJ: Organization of endogenous opiate and nonopiate pain control systems. Science 1982;216:1185–1192.

33   Go VL, Yaksh TL: Release of substance P from the cat spinal cord. J Physiol 1987;391:141–167.

34   Ono H, Mishima A, Ono S, Fukuda H, Vasko MR: Inhibitory effects of clonidine and tizanidine on release of substance P from slices of rat spinal cord and antagonism by alpha-adrenergic receptor antagonists. Neuropharmacology 1991;30:585–589.

35   Fleetwood-Walker SM, Mitchell R, Hope PJ, Molony V, Iggo A: An alpha 2 receptor mediates the selective inhibition by noradrenaline of nociceptive responses of identified dorsal horn neurones. Brain Res 1985;334:243–254.

36   Eisenach JC, Dewan DM, Rose JC, Angelo JM: Epidural clonidine produces antinociception, but not hypotension, in sheep. Anesthesiology 1987;66:496–501.

37   Eisenach JC, Du Pen S, Dubois M, Miguel R, Allin D, and the Epidural Clonidine Study Group: Epidural clonidine analgesia for intractable cancer pain. Pain 1995;61:391–400.

38   Carroll D, Jadad A, King V, Wiffen P, Glynn C, McQuay H: Single-dose, randomized, double-blind, double-dummy, cross-over comparison of extradural and i.v. clonidine in chronic pain. Br J Anaesthesia 1993;71:665–669.

39   Byas-Smith MB, Max MB, Muir J, Kingman A: Transdermal clonidine compared to placebo in painful diabetic neuropathy using a two-stage 'enriched enrollment' design. Pain 1995;60:267–274.

40   Zhuo M, Gebhart GF: Tonic cholinergic inhibition of spinal mechanical transmission. Pain 1991; 46:211–222.

41   Naguib M, Yaksh TL: Antinociceptive effects of spinal cholinesterase inhibition and isobolographic analysis of the interaction with mu and alpha 2 receptor systems. Anesthesiology 1994;80: 1338–1348.

42   Naguib M, Yaksh TL: Characterization of muscarinic receptor subtypes that mediate antinociception in the rat spinal cord. Anesth Analg 1997;85:847–853.

43   Yaksh TL, Dirksen R, Harty GJ: Antinociceptive effects of intrathecally injected cholinomimetic drugs in the rat and car. Eur J Pharmacol 1985;117:81–88.

44   Jänig W, Häbler HJ: Sympathetic nervous system: Contribution to chronic pain. Progr Brain Res 2000;129:451–468.

45   Stanton-Hicks M, Jänig W, Hassenbusch S, Haddox JD, Boas R, Wilson P: Reflex sympathetic dystrophy: Changing concepts and taxonomy. Pain 1995;63:127–133.

46   Harkins SW, Davis MD, Bush FM, Kasberger J: Suppression of first pain and slow temporal summation of second pain in relation to age. J Gerontol A Biol Sci Med Sci 1996;51:M260–M265.

47   Buchtal F, Rosenfalck A: Evoked action potentials and conduction velocity in human sensory nerves. Brain Res 1966;3:1–12.

48   Helme RD, McKernan S: Neurologic flare responses following topical application of capsaicin in humans. Ann Neurol 1985;18:505–509.

49   Parkhouse N, Le Quesne PM: Quantitative objective assessment of peripheral nociceptive C-fibre function. J Neurol Neurosurg Psychiatr 1988;51:28–34.

50   Gagliese L, Melzack R: Age differences in nociception and pain behaviours in the rat. Neurosci Biobehav Rev 2000;24:843–854.

51   Amenta F, Zaccheo D, Collier WL: Neurotransmitters, neuroreceptors and aging. Mech Ageing Dev 1991;61:249–273.

52   Hess GD, Joseph JA, Roth GS: Effect of age on sensitivity to pain and brain opiate receptors. Neurobiol Aging 1981;2:49–55.

53   Missale C, Govoni S, Castelletti L, Spano PF, Trabucchi M: Age related changes of enkephalin in rat spinal cord. Brain Res 1983;262:160–162.

54   Dupont A, Savard P, Merand Y, Labrie F, Boissier JR: Age-related changes in central nervous system enkephalins and substance P. Life Sci 1981;29:2317–2322.

55   Gambert SR, Garthwaite TL, Pontzer CH, Hagen TC: Age-related changes in central nervous system beta-endorphin and ACTH. Neuroendocrinology 1980;31:252–255.

56   Kramer E, Bodnar RJ: Age-related decrements in morphine analgesia: A parametric analysis. Neurobiol Aging 1986;7:185–191.

57   Romero MT, Bodnar RJ: Maintenance of beta-endorphin analgesia across age cohorts. Neurobiol Aging 1987;8:167–170.

58   Bodnar RJ, Romero MT, Kramer E: Organismic variables and pain inhibition: Roles of gender and aging. Brain Res Bull 1988;21:947–953.

59   Hamm RJ, Knisely JS: Environmentally induced analgesia: An age-related decline in an endogenous opioid system. J Gerontol 1985;40:268–274.

60   Guay DRP, Lackner TE, Hanlon JT: Pharmacologic management: Noninvasive modalities; in Weiner DK, Herr K, Rudy TE (eds): Persistent Pain in Older Adults: An Interdisciplinary Guide for Treatment. New York, Springer Publishing Company, 2002, pp 160–187.

61   Hamm RJ, Knisely JS: The analgesia produced by food deprivation in 4-month old, 14-month old, and 24-month old rats. Life Sci 1986;39:1509–1515.

62   Kramer E, Bodnar RJ: Age-related decrements in the analgesic response to cold-water swims. Physiol Behav 1986;36:875–880.

63   Hamm RJ, Knisely JS, Watson A: Environmentally induced analgesia: Age-related differences in a hormonally-mediated, nonopioid system. J Gerontol 1986;41:336–341.

64   Edwards RR, Fillingim RB, Ness TJ: Age-related differences in endogenous pain modulation: A comparison of diffuse noxious inhibitory controls in healthy older and younger adults. Pain 2003;101:155–165.

65   Gibson SJ, Katz B, Corran TM, Farrell MJ, Helme RD: Pain in older persons. Disabil Rehabil 1994;16:127–139.

66   Watkins LR, Katayama Y, Kinscheck IB, Mayer DJ, Hayes RL: Muscarinic cholinergic mediation of opiate and non-opiate environmentally induced analgesias. Brain Res 1984;300:231–242.

67 Knisely JS, Hamm RJ: Physostigmine-induced analgesia in young, middle-aged, and senescent rats. Exp Aging Res 1989;15:3–11.
68 Knisely JS, Hamm RJ: Aging and oxotremorine-induced analgesia. Soc Neurosci Abstr 1985; 11:731.
69 Pedigo NW, Minor LD, Krumrei TN: Cholinergic drug effects and brain muscarinic receptor binding in aged rats. Neurobiol Aging 1984;5:227–233.
70 Chan SH, Lai YY: Effects of aging on pain responses and analgesic efficacy of morphine and clonidine in rats. Exp Neurol 1982;75:112–119.
71 Hamm RJ, Knisely JS: Environmentally induced analgesia: Age-related decline in a neurally mediated, nonopioid system. Psychol Aging 1986;1:195–201.
72 Pascualy M, Petrie EC, Brodkin K, Peskind ER, Veith RC, Raskind MA: Effects of advanced aging on plasma catecholamine responses to the cold pressor test. Neurobiol Aging 1999;20: 637–642.
73 Ramer MS, Bisby MA: Normal and injury-induced sympathetic innervation of rat dorsal root ganglia increases with age. J Comp Neurol 1998;394:38–47.
74 Helgason S, Petursson G, Gudmundsson S, Sigurdsson JA: Prevalence of postherpetic neuralgia after a single episode of herpes zoster: Prospective study with long-term follow-up. Br Med J 2000;321:794–796.
75 Kim YI, Na HS, Yoon YW, Nahm SH, Ko KH, Hong SK: Mechanical allodynia is more strongly manifested in older rats in an experimental model of peripheral neuropathy. Neurosci Lett 1995;199:158–160.
76 Chung JM, Choi Y, Yoon YW, Na HS: Effects of age on behavioral signs of neuropathic pain in an experimental rat model. Neurosci Lett 1995;183:54–57.
77 Tanck EN, Kroin JS, McCarthy RJ, Penn RD, Ivankovich AD: Effects of age and size on development of allodynia in a chronic pain model produced by sciatic nerve ligation in rats. Pain 1992;51:313–316.
78 Ramer MS, Bisby MA: Rapid sprouting of sympathetic axons in dorsal root ganglia of rats with a chronic constriction injury. Pain 1997;70:237–244.
79 Franklin KBJ, Abbott FV: Aging and the neurobiology of pain. Geriatr Aging 2001;4:21–22.

David Lussier, MD
Division of Geriatric Medicine
McGill University Health Center
1650 Cedar Avenue, D17-173
Montreal, Quebec, H3T 1E2 (Canada)
Tel. +1 514 934 8015, Fax +1 514 934 8232, E-Mail david.lussier@muhc.mcgill.ca

Kuchel GA, Hof PR (eds): Autonomic Nervous System in Old Age.
Interdiscipl Top Gerontol. Basel, Karger, 2004, vol 33, pp 120–133

....

Aging and Thermoregulation

R.B. McDonald[a], *A.M. Gabaldón*[b], *B.A. Horwitz*[b]

[a]Department of Nutrition and [b]Section of Neurobiology,
Physiology, and Behavior, University of California, Davis, Calif., USA

Blunted ability to maintain homeothermy has been demonstrated in numerous studies on old laboratory mammals as well as in humans. However, the degree to which this dysfunction reflects the normal biological process of aging in humans is unclear because of confounding effects of extraneous factors. For example, investigators have reported increased death rates in old versus young individuals during periods of excessive heat or cold [1–5]. However, subsequent analysis suggested that adverse socioeconomic factors (i.e., social isolation, lack of air-conditioning/heat) were more important contributors to these deaths than was aging per se [5]. Several of our studies on laboratory rodents have shown that with chronological age, there is generally a modest attenuation of the old animals' ability to maintain homeothermy during several hours of cold exposure, but near the end of life, this attenuation is markedly increased [6–8].

The maintenance of homeothermy involves a complex series of events that have been thoroughly described elsewhere [9, 10]. The biological process of age is an additional influence on these pathways. In humans, the first line of defense against changes in ambient temperature is behavioral (e.g., adding or removing clothes, moving to a less extreme ambient temperature). Laboratory animals also display behavioral changes in response to changing air temperature. Such changes can involve moving to a more 'acceptable' environment or changing position to increase or decrease body heat loss. When behavioral modification fails to maintain appropriate core temperature, peripheral physiological responses will be initiated. During cold exposure, these include vasoconstriction to minimize heat loss, shivering, and nonshivering thermogenesis; during heat exposure, vasodilation, panting, and sweating can be evoked to facilitate loss of body heat. Disruption in any of these processes or their regulation could result in difficulty in maintaining homeothermy.

In this brief review, we will focus on how aging alters the various processes that contribute to effective thermoregulation. Although age-related changes to thermoregulatory responses of older humans are a primary concern, most of the mechanistic studies have used rodents as model systems. This is especially true for responses to cold exposure. Thus, our discussion on age-related alterations to heat exposure will focus on humans whereas responses to cold will include both human and laboratory animals.

Heat-Induced Reponses in the Elderly

Epidemiological data have suggested that individuals over the age of 70 years are more susceptible to heat exposure than are young people [2, 3]. However, subsequent analyses of these data sets found that living conditions and/or underlying disease contributed significantly to this attenuated heat tolerance and perhaps more so than did chronological age. For example, Mirchandani et al. [5] reported that in 1993, the heat-related deaths of elderly individuals living alone in Philadelphia without air conditioning were more related to their pre-existing disease state than to their age. Additionally, imprecise measurement of core temperature, lack of data on hydration state of the individual, reliance on medical record data, and overinterpretation of cross-sectional analyses have confounded the conclusion that heat tolerance is diminished in the elderly. Although some human data suggest that age-related decreases in heat tolerance are related to modifiable environmental factors, other data indicate that the elderly do exhibit physiological alterations of individual components of heat dissipation mechanisms (i.e., sweat rate, skin blood flow, and cardiovascular adjustments) [11–13].

The cooling effect of sweat evaporation contributes significantly to maintenance of homeothermy during heat exposure, and several investigators have proposed that decreased sweat rates of older versus younger individuals may explain, at least partially, their differences in response to a heat challenge [11, 14–16]. Some studies using localized injections of the cholinergic analog methylcholine to increase sweating have noted age-related attenuation in sweat rates with no significant differences in sweat gland density [17]. Others, using the same methodology for inducing sweating, have not always found differences with age. Inoue [15] and Inoue et al. [18] suggest that such inconsistencies may largely reflect the different anatomical sites being studied. In a five-year longitudinal investigation of older men, Inoue [15] found that total sweat rates significantly decreased over time, while changes in site-specific sweat rates varied with the site, some decreasing, some increasing, and some remaining unchanged. Thus, depending on the anatomical area, sweat gland density and/or output per gland may be blunted with age.

Two other important mechanisms for coping with heat exposure involve the cardiovascular system. One of these is the redirection of cardiac output from the body core to the skin; the other is dilation of peripheral blood vessels (vasodilation). Although some studies have reported no effect of age on cardiac output [19, 20], Kenney et al. [21] found lower cardiac outputs and lower heart rates in older men (61–73 years of age) exercising in the heat at intensities up to 60% $VO_{2,max}$ than in younger subjects (21–33 years of age). Kenney and Zappe [13] have also reported that the redistribution of total cardiac output from splanchnic and renal beds to the skin was less in older versus younger individuals despite the fact that both groups were exercising at matched intensities in a warm environment (30°C) [13]. This attenuation would be expected to result in less heat lost from the skin.

Data related to altered age-related skin blood flow during heat exposure are more consistent than cardiac output data. A series of investigations by Kenney et al. [21, 22] and Kenney and Armstrong [23] led them to conclude that skin blood flow at a given core temperature during passive (non-exertion-induced) and active (exercise-induced) heat stress is significantly lower in older than in younger subjects as a result of altered cutaneous vasodilation. That is, resistance to flow, as measured by occlusion plethysmography and laser Doppler flowmetry, was significantly greater in their older versus younger subjects following skin warming. (For a more detailed review of these experiments, see Horwitz et al. [24].) Moreover, this age-related attenuated vasodilation appears to involve nitric oxide- as well as axon reflex-mediated mechanisms [25, 26]. Thus, the data from Kenney's lab support the view that decreased cardiac output, less effective redistribution of blood flow to the skin, and reduced cutaneous vasodilation may all contribute to the attenuated heat tolerance of old individuals.

This conclusion notwithstanding, it is important to note that one factor that is not always considered when documenting the response of the elderly to heat is their acclimation state. Studies matching young and old subjects with respect to levels of heat acclimation, body composition and/or physical fitness suggest that these factors may be as important or more so to the ability to maintain homeothermy during heat exposure than is age [20]. Indeed, Yousef et al. [20] noted that young and old men and women who were matched for heat acclimation had similar rectal and skin temperatures, heart rates, and total sweat loss after a 1-hour desert walk (40–44°C) at a work intensity of 40% $VO_{2,max}$. Thus, at least in some cases, age-related diminution of heat tolerance may be associated with 'disuse' rather than aging per se.

Aging and Cold-Induced Thermoregulation

The physiological processes that allow maintenance of homeothermy during cold exposure involve a complex series of regulatory steps and have been described thoroughly elsewhere [24]. Briefly, when exposed to temperatures below thermoneutrality (temperature of thermoneutrality varies with the species), thermoreceptors in the skin, spinal cord, and brain transmit neural signals to the hypothalamus. In a process that is not completely understood, the hypothalamus integrates this information and initiates neural signals to the periphery that result in decreased heat loss and increased heat production. Heat loss is minimized by increasing cutaneous vasoconstriction, while heat production is increased as a result of shivering in skeletal muscle and nonshivering thermogenic processes in brown adipose tissue and to a lesser degree, in other tissues. Failure of this integrated system to conserve core temperature results in hypothermia, and severe hypothermia may lead to cardio-insufficiency and death.

Several investigations have reported age-related increases in morbidity and mortality of individuals exposed to extended periods of excessive cold [1, 4, 27]. Similar to investigations describing blunted thermoregulation during heat exposure, data supporting attenuated cold-induced thermoregulation in the elderly are confounded by numerous variables. Among these are underlying disease, physical fitness, cold acclimation, and factors related to socioeconomic status [28]. Nonetheless, a greater susceptibility to cold is consistent with the finding that 9% of the elderly in the United Kingdom had morning core temperatures within 0.5°C of the clinical definition of hypothermia, 35°C [29].

The ability to appropriately thermoregulate in the cold is dependent on accurate cold perception. Behavioral studies have suggested that the perception of decreasing ambient temperature is significantly impaired in older versus younger subjects [1]. For example, when similarly dressed young and old subjects were placed in a 19°C room and asked to manually adjust the room temperature to their comfort zone, elderly individuals exhibited less precise control as reflected by a greater amplitude of oscillations in their adjusted temperatures over the 2.5-hour exposure period. When these same individuals were asked to discriminate between close temperature differences, the younger men were able to distinguish ambient temperature changes of approximately 1.0°C, whereas some older subjects were unable to detect differences less than 2°C [1]. Along similar lines, Watts [30] found that some older women felt cold only at relatively low ambient temperatures.

Thermoregulatory heat production via shivering and nonshivering thermogenesis is critical to the overall maintenance of core temperature during cold exposure. Since skeletal muscle shivering is the major source of cold-induced heat production in humans and other large mammals, and several studies have reported significant declines in lean body mass of elderly humans [for a review, see ref. 31], it is not surprising that investigators have focused on blunted shivering thermogenesis as a possible cause of the elderly's cold-induced hypothermia. Although elderly individuals retain the ability for shivering, there is evidence that their onset of shivering during cold exposure is delayed compared to that of younger individuals [32]. Moreover, some studies have shown that the intensity of shivering, as measured by peak contractile strength, is significantly less in the old versus young subjects [33, 34], suggesting attenuated heat production. Age-related disruption in shivering thermogenesis may also reflect reduced metabolic capacity of muscle cells. Impaired glucose uptake into the muscle of insulin-resistant older individuals could reduce shivering during cold exposure [35, 36], although direct evidence for this effect is limited [37]. Others report that the reduced shivering thermogenesis of old versus young subjects may closely reflect decreased activity of skeletal muscle enzymes involved in aerobic metabolism – enzymes such as succinate dehydrogenase, malate dehydrogenase, and citrate synthase [38–40]. However, other research indicates that age-related alterations in muscle metabolic capacity may be associated more with a sedentary lifestyle than with aging per se [41, 42].

Heat conservation mechanisms also play a primary role in the ability to maintain body temperature during exposure to cold. Decreased skin blood flow and decreased peripheral vasoconstriction represent two major contributors to heat conservation in mammals, and some investigations have suggested that these mechanisms are altered in aging. For example, in a longitudinal study of 43 elderly males, Collins et al. [27] found that the number who showed no cold-induced decrease in hand blood flow rose from 14% (6) to 32.5% (14) 4 years later and was further increased 8 years after the study began. Although other studies evaluating cutaneous fingertip blood flow as an index of vascular constriction during cold exposure suggest a similar magnitude of cold-induced vasoconstriction in young and old subjects [43], there is some indication that attaining maximal vasoconstriction takes longer in the elderly than in younger subjects [44]. In addition, this vasoconstriction may not be retained as long in the elderly. Richardson et al. [44] found that although cold-induced vasoconstriction occurred within the first minute in both young and old subjects, the response was not maintained in the latter, and blood flow returned to pre-cold levels before the cold exposure was terminated.

Reduced cold-induced vasoconstriction in the peripheral vasculature could result from altered arterial wall stiffness and/or altered neural and hormonal stimuli. With respect to the former, greater vessel diameter and wall thickness have been associated with age-related increases in arterial wall stiffness [45]. However, most investigations reporting increased arterial wall stiffness have focused on large vessels due primarily to ease of measurement. It is not clear whether similar increases in vessel wall stiffness occur in the smaller vessels innervating the skin, i.e., those primarily responsible for heat conservation.

Similarly, the jury is still out on the physiological importance of any altered hormonal/neural modulation of vasoconstriction with age. Hogikyan and Supiano [46] have reported that blunted skin vasoconstriction, as measured during α-adrenergic stimulation, is slightly reduced in older versus younger subjects, but total blood flow is not. These investigators concluded that increased sympathetic neural signaling compensated for the altered α-adrenergic responsiveness of the older subjects. Clearly, additional studies are required to fully understand the mechanism underlying diminished vasoconstriction responsiveness during cold exposure of the elderly.

Thermoregulation in Cold-Exposed Aging Rodents

Human studies describing age-related differences in cold tolerance are limited by the difficulties in performing longitudinal studies with significant numbers of individuals as well as the inability to utilize invasive techniques to study underlying mechanisms. These constraints have led to the widespread use of laboratory rodents for studies focusing on mechanisms. Although most of these studies have utilized a cross-sectional rather than a longitudinal design, they have provided insight into changes that occur with age. As with the data from humans, there are factors that can significantly affect the results. Among these are gender, rodent strain, diet, physical fitness, temperature of acclimation, and length and intensity of the cold exposure. The age of the groups being compared is also important. Because rats and mice undergo relatively rapid growth/development until they are about 4 months old, comparisons using animals younger than 4 months of age make it difficult to determine whether their differences with older rodents reflect development or aging. By the same token, data from 'old' rodents that are significantly younger than the median life span for the strain can lead to spurious interpretations. Notwithstanding all of these caveats, results from a number of investigators demonstrate that, like humans, the maintenance of homeothermy during cold exposure is less robust in old versus young rodents [24, 47].

In terms of mechanisms, the available evidence supports the view that the failure of cold-exposed old rodents to maintain homeothermy is more attributable to age-related changes in heat generation than in heat conservation. With respect to the latter, body composition studies of several rat strains have shown little or no decrease in percent carcass fat in old versus young rats [6, 48–51]. These data suggest that there is no significant diminution of the insulative capacity of older rats due to less adipose tissue. There also does not appear to be a loss in the ability to vasoconstrict peripheral blood vessels when the animals are cold exposed. In fact, some studies have suggested that older mice and rats have more robust vasoconstriction than younger animals [52–55]. This greater vasoconstrictor response of the cold-exposed older rodents may compensate for their reduced heat generation. Thus, while in some cases there may be changes in the insulative properties of the fur, there is little evidence that physiological mechanisms associated with vasoconstrictor responses are diminished with chronological age.

The same appears to be true for behavioral mechanisms associated with thermoregulation. The preferred temperature of old F344 male rats does not differ significantly from that of younger animals [56]. Moreover, both young and old Sprague-Dawley rats have been shown to work equally well for heat by pressing a lever that turned on a heat lamp [57].

In contrast, several (although not all) studies have observed attenuated heat production in cold-exposed older rats and mice. This attenuation may involve reduced shivering as well as reduced nonshivering thermogenesis, at least in some rodent strains. Evidence for an involvement of shivering comes from indirect, rather than direct, observations. For example, older mammals often have less muscle mass and less skeletal muscle oxidative capacity, both of which would reduce the maximum amount of heat able to be generated by skeletal muscle cells [31]. Based on their studies with Sprague-Dawley male rats, Lee and Wang [58] and Wang et al. [59] have suggested that substrate for cold-induced muscle heat production is less available in old versus young rats, thus limiting the amount of thermogenesis that can be achieved through shivering.

Substrate limitation does not appear to occur in brown adipose tissue, the major site of cold-induced nonshivering heat production in rodents [58]. Although brown fat generates relatively little heat in adult humans as compared to the heat generated via shivering [60, 61], it remains an important source of thermogenesis in adult mice and rats [62]. Many of the events involved in brown fat heat production have been identified and are discussed at length elsewhere [63]. Briefly, during cold exposure, hypothalamic signaling results in activation of the sympathetic nervous system and transmission of signals to brown adipose tissue. Norepinephrine, released at the brown adipocytes binds to both α- and β-adrenergic receptors, but it is the latter interaction that plays the major role in initiating the ensuing thermogenesis. Binding of norepinephrine to β_3-receptors activates the G-protein-adenylyl cyclase-cAMP pathway that leads to phosphorylation of hormone-sensitive lipase and enhanced hydrolysis of intracellular triacylglycerides. The resulting fatty acids not only serve as substrate for mitochondrial oxidative metabolism, they also activate molecules of uncoupling protein-1 (UCP1) in the inner mitochondrial membrane. This, in turn, promotes the transfer of protons back into the mitochondrial matrix, thereby dissipating the driving force for ATP synthesis and stimulating the rate of fatty acid oxidation. As a result, more fatty acids are oxidized and more heat is generated than would be the case if the mitochondria remained coupled.

The total heat-producing potential of brown adipose tissue is directly related to the number of brown adipocytes and the UCP1 concentration within each adipocyte. Rodents with large depots of brown fat (relative to body mass) tend to have greater resistance to the development of hypothermia during cold exposure. Cross-sectional studies on rats and mice housed in thermoneutrality have shown that brown fat depots decrease in mass with age as do total protein and UCP1 concentrations. Consistent with this decrease is the fact that old rodents not only exhibit greater hypothermia during cold exposure than do their younger counterparts [50–52, 64–67] they also exhibit blunted cold-induced oxygen consumption (heat production) and blunted norepinephrine-induced oxygen consumption [50, 52, 58, 68]. Thus, at least part of the age-related decline in the cold-induced thermogenesis of older rodents may be attributable to the presence of fewer thermogenically active brown adipocytes [51].

Another possibility that has been examined is that sympathetic signaling to brown fat is diminished in the cold-exposed older (versus younger) rats. We tested this hypothesis by evaluating brown fat norepinephrine turnover at rest and during cold exposure in 6-, 12- and 26-month-old male and female F344 rats [8]. We found that cold exposure enhanced norepinephrine turnover in all age groups and genders. Interestingly, the group with the lowest core temperature during the 2 h of cold exposure (i.e., 26-month-old male rats) had the greatest brown fat norepinephrine turnover, indicating appropriate neural signaling. Kawate et al. [69] also reported that sympathetic signaling to brown fat of aged (30 months) and young (10 months) C57BL/6J mice, as measured by direct neural recording, was greater in the older animals. These data demonstrate that the thermoregulatory pathway from thermoreceptor to hypothalamus to sympathetic signaling remains intact in the older rodents, and neural signaling to brown adipose tissue of old rodents is not attenuated.

Although sympathetic signaling may remain robust in older animals, reduction in brown adipocyte beta–receptor number could contribute to decreased thermogenesis. There is evidence that brown fat β_1- and β_2-adrenergic receptor number and responsiveness decline significantly with age. Scarpace et al. [70] reported an age-related decrease in receptor density associated with reduced adenylyl cyclase activity, suggesting both blunted receptor function and postreceptor signaling. However, our data indicate that brown adipocytes isolated from old rats are not less responsive to sympathetic stimulation than are cells isolated from young rats [71]. That is, norepinephrine elicited similar dose-dependent increases in oxygen consumption of cells from young and old male and female F344 rats; there were no effects of age or gender on values of V_{max} or EC_{50} (the concentration of agent eliciting one half of V_{max}). Moreover, we found no significant differences in oxygen consumption among the age and gender groups when isolated adipocytes were exposed to a single dose of the

β_3-adrenergic agonist, CL-316,243. Therefore, even if there were age-related declines in β-adrenergic density or binding, they did not translate into less brown adipocyte thermogenesis.

These data suggest that neither reduced sympathetic signaling or reduced responsiveness of brown adipocytes can explain the blunted cold-induced thermogenesis of old rodents. This attenuation appears to be more closely associated with the presence of less brown adipose tissue, suggesting that the ability of preadipocytes to proliferate and mature into thermogenically functional brown adipocytes is diminished with age.

Effect of Gender on Cold-Induced Thermoregulatory Responses

Data from humans indicate that hypothermia is more prevalent in elderly men than in elderly women [5, 72, 73]. Consistent with these findings are our observations of gender differences with respect to the effects of age on cold-induced thermoregulatory responses of F344 rats [64]. Our studies clearly show that older male rats are more susceptible to hypothermia than are comparably aged females exposed to cold for identical periods of time [51, 64]. Part of this increased susceptibility may reflect the fact that old female rats generally have a higher percentage of carcass fat than do old males [51]. In addition, brown fat thermogenesis appears to be lower in cold-exposed old male versus female rats because the males have less functional brown fat than the females. That is, brown fat depots in older F344 male rats weigh less and have less protein, lower levels of UCP1, and less cold-induced glucose utilization than depots of brown fat of similarly aged female rats [64, 74]. This gender difference in brown fat metabolism (i.e., glucose utilization) of the cold-exposed old rats is not due to less sympathetic stimulation in the males, as evidenced by the fact that their brown fat norepinephrine turnover is greater than that of the females [8]. Moreover, as described above, brown adipocytes isolated from old male and female rats respond comparably to norepinephrine stimulation [71]. Thus, the lower in vivo metabolic activity of brown fat in cold-exposed old males versus females is most likely due to the presence of fewer thermogenically active brown adipocytes. The basis for this gender difference in the number of brown adipocytes has not been delineated.

Senescence and Thermoregulation in Rats

In the course of our investigations we serendipitously observed that the greatest magnitude of hypothermia in a group of cold-exposed aged rats occurred in animals that weighed the least. Further inspection of our longitudinal data collected from rats fed ad libitum indicated that older rats appeared to undergo a rapid and spontaneous weight loss near the end of life, a condition that is known to also occur in humans [75]. These data suggested that the animals exhibiting rapid spontaneous weight loss may have entered a thermoregulatory dysfunctional state. To test this hypothesis, we exposed male F344 rats to 6°C for 4h every 14 days beginning at 24 months of age (median life span of F344 rats being ~25.5 months) and until the onset of rapid spontaneous weight loss [7]. All rats displaying spontaneous rapid weight loss (rats that we refer to as senescent) became significantly more hypothermic during the acute cold exposure than they did before exhibiting the weight loss. Moreover, weight-stable rats of identical age were able to maintain a relatively normal core temperature during cold exposure. To determine whether this increased susceptibility to hypothermia resulted from the weight loss of the senescent rats, we measured the responses of 26-month-old presenescent animals (weight stable) that were food restricted to same weight loss as the senescent rats. When these food-restricted presenescent rats were exposed to cold under the same conditions as the senescent rats, they did not develop severe hypothermia [7]. Thus, the body weight loss of the senescent rats is an indicator that the rats had entered a different functional state rather than being the cause of this state. Interestingly, the start of the rapid and spontaneous weight loss did not correlate with chronological age. The age at which rats entered this phase varied from 24 to 30 months and could not be predicted from behavioral or physiological measurements at earlier ages.

Further studies have shown that not only do senescent rats exhibit altered feeding behavior [76] and decreased ability to maintain homeothermy [7], they also have disrupted circadian rhythms of body temperature [77]. When we measured the endogenous (i.e., under constant dark condition) circadian rhythm of body temperature in aging rats during their presenescent and senescent periods as well as in young (10 month) rats, we observed significant disruption of this rhythm in the senescent animals [77]. The fact that this disruption occurred near the onset of senescence when regulation of feeding and cold-induced thermoregulation (processes involving hypothalamic regulation) were also adversely affected strongly suggests that the early stages of senescence involve alterations in hypothalamic regulation.

Conclusions

Investigations using humans have shown that the incidence of hyper- and hypothermia increases with age. These studies are confounded, however, by potential differences in physical fitness, socioeconomic status, disease, and prior heat or cold acclimation. Thus, it is not clear whether altered thermoregulation, as suggested by human studies, is the result of aging per se or of other factors that have an impact on normal physiology. Nonetheless, investigations evaluating selected components of the thermoregulatory system have described significant alterations in healthy aging subjects. These include altered sweat gland function, vasodilation and vasoconstriction, temperature perception, and skin blood flow. Clearly, the full elucidation of the effects that aging has on human thermoregulation will require significantly more research.

Although studies of age-related changes in thermoregulatory responses of rodents provide a means whereby extraneous variables can be more precisely controlled, mechanisms underlying the decreased ability to maintain homeothermy have yet to be fully identified. Alterations in brown fat thermogenesis, body composition, and hypothalamic regulation have all been identified as possible contributors. However, these changes do not occur in all rodents, are modulated by gender, and are not tightly correlated with chronological age. Initial studies on neurotransmitter changes in the central nervous system of aged rats are opening the way for more complete evaluation of the effects of aging on regulation of physiological processes such as thermoregulation. The rat is an excellent model for future neural studies on the hierarchical thermoregulatory system, an area as yet relatively unexplored in aging research; and transgenic mice offer the possibility of testing the role of candidate genes modulating age-related changes in thermal responses.

Acknowledgements

We thank Jock Hamilton for his assistance in the preparation of the manuscript. Research from our laboratories has been funded by NIA Grant AG06665 and a gift from the California Age Research Institute.

References

1   Collins KJ, Exton-Smith AN, Dore C: Urban hypothermia: Preferred temperature and thermal perception in old age. Br Med J (Clin Res Ed) 1981;282:175–177.
2   Levine JA: Heat stroke in the aged. Am J Med 1969;47:251–258.
3   Lye M, Kamal A: Effects of a heat wave on mortality rates in elderly inpatients. Lancet 1977;i:529–531.
4   Macey SM, Schneider DF: Deaths from excessive heat and excessive cold among the elderly. Gerontologist 1993;33:497–500.
5   Mirchandani HG, McDonald G, Hood IC, Fonseca C: Heat-related deaths in Philadelphia–1993. Am J Forensic Med Pathol 1996;17:106–108.
6   McDonald RB, Stern JS, Horwitz B: Cold-induced metabolism and brown fat GDP binding in young and old rats. Exp Gerontol 1987;22:409–420.

7   McDonald RB, Florez-Duquet M, Murtagh-Mark C, Horwitz BA: Relationship between cold-induced thermoregulation and spontaneous rapid body weight loss of aging F344 rats. Am J Physiol 1996;271:R1115–R1122.

8   McDonald RB, Hamilton JS, Horwitz BA: Influence of age and gender on brown adipose tissue norepinephrine turnover. Proc Soc Exp Biol Med 1993;204:117–121.

9   Gordon CJ: Thermal biology of the laboratory rat. Physiol Behav 1990;47:963–991.

10   Rothwell NJ: CNS regulation of thermogenesis. Crit Rev Neurobiol 1994;8:1–10.

11   Fennell WH, Moore RE: Responses of aged men to passive heating. J Physiol 1973;231:118P–119P.

12   Kenney WL: Thermoregulation at rest and during exercise in healthy older adults. Exerc Sport Sci Rev 1997;25:41–76.

13   Kenney WL, Zappe DH: Effect of age on renal blood flow during exercise. Aging (Milano) 1994; 6:293–302.

14   Crowe JP, Moore RE: Proceedings: Physiological and behavioral responses of aged men to passive heating. J Physiol 1974;236:43P–45P.

15   Inoue Y: Longitudinal effects of age on heat-activated sweat gland density and output in healthy active older men. Eur J Appl Physiol Occup Physiol 1996;74:72–77.

16   Shoenfeld Y, Udassin R, Shapiro Y, Ohri A, Sohar E: Age and sex difference in response to short exposure to extreme dry heat. J Appl Physiol 1978;44:1–4.

17   Kenney WL, Fowler SR: Methylcholine-activated eccrine sweat gland density and output as a function of age. J Appl Physiol 1988;65:1082–1086.

18   Inoue Y, Nakao M, Okudaira S, Ueda H, Araki T: Seasonal variation in sweating responses of older and younger men. Eur J Appl Physiol Occup Physiol 1995;70:6–12.

19   Sawka MN: Physiological responses to acute exercise heat stress; in Pandolf KB, Sawka MN, Gonzalez RR (eds): Human Performance Physiology and Environmental Medicine at Terrestrial Extremes. Indianapolis, Benchmark Press, 1988, p 637.

20   Yousef MK, Dill DB, Vitez TS, Hillyard SD, Goldman AS: Thermoregulatory responses to desert heat: Age, race and sex. J Gerontol 1984;39:406–414.

21   Kenney WL, Morgan AL, Farquhar WB, Brooks EM, Pierzga JM, Derr JA: Decreased active vasodilator sensitivity in aged skin. Am J Physiol 1997;272:H1609–H1614.

22   Kenney WL, Tankersley CG, Newswanger DL, Puhl SM: Alpha-1-adrenergic blockade does not alter control of skin blood flow during exercise. Am J Physiol 1991;260:H855–H861.

23   Kenney WL, Armstrong CG: Reflex peripheral vasoconstriction is diminished in older men. J Appl Physiol 1996;80:512–515.

24   Horwitz BA, Gabaldón AM, McDonald RM: Thermoregulation during aging; in Hof PR, Mobbs CV (eds): Functional Neurobiology of Aging. San Diego, Academic Press, 2001, pp 839–854.

25   Minson CT, Holowatz LA, Wong BJ, Kenney WL, Wilkins BW: Decreased nitric oxide- and axon reflex-mediated cutaneous vasodilation with age during local heating. J Appl Physiol 2002;93: 1644–1649.

26   Holowatz LA, Houghton B, Wong BJ, Wilkins BW, Harding AW, Kenney WL, Minson CT: Nitric oxide and attenuated reflex cutaneous vasodilation in aged skin. Am J Physiol Heart Circ Physiol 2003;284:H1662–H1667.

27   Collins KJ, Dore C, Exton-Smith AN, Fox RH, MacDonald IC, Woodward PM: Accidental hypothermia and impaired temperature homoeostasis in the elderly. Br Med J 1977;1:353–356.

28   Young AJ: Effects of aging on human cold tolerance. Exp Aging Res 1991;17:205–213.

29   Collins KJ: Effects of cold on old people. Br J Hosp Med 1987;38:506–514.

30   Watts AJ: Hypothermia in the aged: A study of the role of cold-sensitivity. Environ Res 1972; 5:119–126.

31   McCarter RJM: Energy utilization; in Masoro EJ (ed): Aging: Handbook of Physiology, section 11. New York, Oxford University Press, 1995, pp 95–118.

32   Kenney WL, Buskirk ER: Functional consequences of sarcopenia: Effects on thermoregulation. J Gerontol A Biol Sci Med Sci 1995;50(Spec No):78–85.

33   Horvath SM, Radcliffe CE, Hutt BK, Spurr GB: Metabolic responses of old people to a cold environment. J Appl Physiol 1955;8:145–148.

34   Wagner JA, Robinson S, Marino RP: Age and temperature regulation of humans in neutral and cold environments. J Appl Physiol 1974;37:562–565.

35 Defronzo RA: Glucose intolerance and aging. Diabetes 1979;28:1095–1101.
36 Reaven GM, Chen N, Hollenbeck C, Chen Y-DI: Effect of age on glucose tolerance and glucose uptake in healthy individuals: J Am Geriatr Soc 1989;37:735–740.
37 Buemann BA, Astrup A, Christensen NJ, Madsen J: Effect of moderate cold exposure on 24-h expenditure: Similar response in postobese and nonobese women. Am J Physiol 1992;263: E1040–E1045.
38 Coggan AR, Spina RJ, King DS, Rogers MA, Brown M, Nemeth PM, Holloszy JO: Histochemical and enzymatic comparison of the gastrocnemius muscle of young and elderly men and women. J Gerontol 1992;47:B71–B76.
39 Ermini M: Ageing changes in mammalian skeletal muscle: Biochemical studies. Gerontology 1976;22:301–316.
40 Essen-Gustavsson B, Borges O: Histochemical and metabolic characteristics of human skeletal muscle in relation to age. Acta Physiol Scand 1986;126:107–114.
41 Coggan AR, Spina RJ, King DS, Rogers MA, Brown M, Nemeth PM, Holloszy JO: Histochemical and enzymatic characteristics of skeletal muscle in master athletes. J Appl Physiol 1990;68: 1896–1901.
42 Proctor DN, Sinning WE, Walro JM, Sieck GC, Lemon PWR: Oxidative capacity of human muscle fiber types: Effects of age and training status. J Appl Physiol 1995;78:2033–2038.
43 Khan F, Spence VA, Belch JJF: Cutaneous vascular responses and thermoregulation in relation to age. Clin Sci 1992;82:521–528.
44 Richardson D, Tyra J, McCray A: Attenuation of the cutaneous vasoconstrictor response to cold in elderly men. J Gerontol A Biol Sci Med Sci 1992;47:M211–M214.
45 Lakatta EB: Cardiovascular system; in Masoro EJ (ed): Handbook of Physiology, section 11: Aging. New York, Oxford University Press, 1995, pp 413–474.
46 Hogikyan RV, Supiano MA: Arterial α-adrenergic responsiveness is decreased and SNS activity is increased in older humans. Am J Physiol 1994;266:E717–E724.
47 Florez-Duquet M, McDonald RB: Cold-induced thermoregulation and biological aging. Physiol Rev 1998;78:339–358.
48 McDonald RB, Stern JS, Horwitz BA: Thermogenic responses of younger and older rats to cold exposure: Comparison of two strains. J Gerontol 1989;44:B37–B42.
49 McDonald RB, Horwitz BA, Stern JS: Cold-induced thermogenesis in younger and older Fischer 344 rats following exercise training. Am J Physiol 1988;254:R908–R916.
50 McDonald RB, Horwitz BA, Hamilton JS, Stern JS: Cold- and norepinephrine-induced thermogenesis in younger and older Fischer 344 rats. Am J Physiol 1988;254:R457–R462.
51 McDonald RB, Day C, Carlson K, Stern JS, Horwitz BA: Effect of age and gender on thermoregulation. Am J Physiol 1989;257:R700–R704.
52 Balmagiya T, Rozovski SJ: Age-related changes in thermoregulation in male albino rats. Exp Gerontol 1983;18:199–210.
53 Cox B, Lee TF, Parkes J: Decreased ability to cope with heat and cold linked to a dysfunction in a central dopaminergic pathway in elderly rats. Life Sci 1981;28:2039–2044.
54 Talan MI: Age-related changes in thermoregulation of mice. Ann N Y Acad Sci 1997;813:95–100.
55 Schaefer VI, Talan MI, Shechtman O: The effect of exercise training on cold tolerance in adult and old C57BL/6J mice. J Gerontol A Biol Sci Med Sci 1996;51:B38–B42.
56 Owen TL, Spencer RL, Duckles SP: Effect of age on cold acclimation in rats: Metabolic and behavioral responses. Am J Physiol 1991;260:R284–R289.
57 Jakubczak LF: Behavioral thermoregulation in young and old rats. J Appl Physiol 1966;21:19–21.
58 Lee TF, Wang LC: Improving cold tolerance in elderly rats by aminophylline. Life Sci 1985;36: 2025–2032.
59 Wang LC, Jin ZL, Lee TF: Decrease in cold tolerance of aged rats caused by the enhanced endogenous adenosine activity. Pharmacol Biochem Behav 1992;43:117–123.
60 Heaton JM: The distribution of brown adipose tissue in the human. J Anat 1972;112:35–39.
61 Ito T, Tanuma Y, Yamada M, Yamamoto M: Morphological studies on brown adipose tissue in the bat and in humans of various ages. Arch Histol Cytol 1991;54:1–39.
62 Foster DO, Frydman ML: Tissue distribution of cold-induced thermogenesis in conscious warm- or cold-acclimated rats reevaluated from changes in tissue blood flow: The dominant role of brown

adipose tissue in the replacement of shivering by nonshivering thermogenesis. Can J Physiol Pharmacol 1979;57:257–270.

63   Himms-Hagen J: The role of brown adipose tissue thermogenesis in energy balance; in Cryere A, Van RLR (eds): New Perspectives in Adipose Tissue: Structure, Function and Development. London, Buttorworths, 1985, pp 199–222.

64   Gabaldón AM, Florez-Duquet ML, Hamilton JS, McDonald RB, Horwitz BA: Effects of age and gender on brown fat and skeletal muscle metabolic responses to cold in F344 rats. Am J Physiol 1995;268:R931–R941.

65   Hoffman-Goetz L, Keir R: Body temperature responses of aged mice to ambient temperature and humidity stress. J Gerontol 1984;39:547–551.

66   Scarpace PJ: Thermoregulation with age: Role of beta-adrenergic signal transduction. Ann N Y Acad Sci 1997;813:111–116.

67   Talan MI, Engel BT, Whitaker JR: A longitudinal study of tolerance to cold stress among C57BL/6J mice. J Gerontol 1985;40:8–14.

68   Kiang-Ulrich M, Horvath SM: Age-related differences in response to acute cold challenge (−10 degrees C) in male F344 rats. Exp Gerontol 1985;20:201–209.

69   Kawate R, Talan MI, Engel BT: Aged C57BL/6J mice respond to cold with increased sympathetic nervous activity in interscapular brown adipose tissue. J Gerontol 1993;48:B180–B183.

70   Scarpace PJ, Mooradian AD, Morley JE: Age-associated decrease in beta-adrenergic receptors and adenylate cyclase activity in rat brown adipose tissue. J Gerontol 1988;43:B65–B70.

71   Gabaldón AM, McDonald RB, Horwitz BA: Effects of age, gender, and senescence on beta-adrenergic responses of isolated F344 rat brown adipocytes in vitro. Am J Physiol 1998;274: E726–E736.

72   Wagner JA, Horvath SM: Cardiovascular reactions to cold exposures differ with age and gender. J Appl Physiol 1985;58:187–192.

73   Wagner JA, Horvath SM: Influences of age and gender on human thermoregulatory responses to cold exposures. J Appl Physiol 1985;58:180–186.

74   McDonald RB, Murtagh CM, Horwitz BA: Age and gender effects on glucose utilization in skeletal muscle and brown adipose tissue of cold-exposed rats. Proc Soc Exp Biol Med 1994;207: 102–109.

75   Sarkisian CA, Lachs MS: Failure to thrive in older adults. Ann Intern Med 1996;124:1072–1078.

76   Blanton CA, Horwitz BA, Murtagh-Mark C, Gietzen DW, Griffey SM, McDonald RB: Meal patterns associated with the age-related decline in food intake in the Fischer 344 rat. Am J Physiol 1998;275:R1494–R1502.

77   McDonald RB, Hoban-Higgins TM, Ruhe RC, Fuller CA, Horwitz BA: Alterations in endogenous circadian rhythm of core temperature in senescent Fischer 344 rats. Am J Physiol 1999;276: R824–R830.

B. A. Horwitz
Neurobiology, Physiology, & Behavior, University of California
One Shields Ave., Davis, CA 95616 (USA)
Tel. +1 530 752 2072, Fax +1 530 752 6359, E-Mail bahorwitz@ucdavis.edu

Author Index

Subject Index